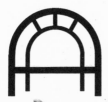

THE ALTRUISTIC BRAIN

THE ALTRUISTIC BRAIN

How We Are Naturally Good

DONALD W. PFAFF, PhD

WITH

SANDRA SHERMAN

OXFORD
UNIVERSITY PRESS

OXFORD
UNIVERSITY PRESS

Oxford University Press is a department of the University of
Oxford. It furthers the University's objective of excellence in research,
scholarship, and education by publishing worldwide.

Oxford   New York
Auckland   Cape Town   Dar es Salaam   Hong Kong   Karachi
Kuala Lumpur   Madrid   Melbourne   Mexico City   Nairobi
New Delhi   Shanghai   Taipei   Toronto

With offices in
Argentina   Austria   Brazil   Chile   Czech Republic   France   Greece
Guatemala   Hungary   Italy   Japan   Poland   Portugal   Singapore
South Korea   Switzerland   Thailand   Turkey   Ukraine   Vietnam

Oxford is a registered trademark of Oxford University Press
in the UK and certain other countries.

Published in the United States of America by
Oxford University Press
198 Madison Avenue, New York, NY 10016

Library of Congress Cataloging-in-Publication Data
Pfaff, Donald W., 1939–author.
The altruistic brain : how we are naturally good / Donald Pfaff.
    p. ; cm.
Includes bibliographical references and index.
ISBN 978–0–19–937746–6 (alk. paper)
I. Title.
[DNLM: 1. Altruism.   2. Brain—physiology.   3. Behavior—physiology.
4. Biological Evolution. WL 337]
BF637.H4
155.2′32—dc23
2014012452

The science of medicine is a rapidly changing field. As new research and clinical experience broaden our
knowledge, changes in treatment and drug therapy occur. The author and publisher of this work have
checked with sources believed to be reliable in their efforts to provide information that is accurate and
complete, and in accordance with the standards accepted at the time of publication. However, in light of
the possibility of human error or changes in the practice of medicine, neither the author, nor the publisher,
nor any other party who has been involved in the preparation or publication of this work warrants that the
information contained herein is in every respect accurate or complete. Readers are encouraged to confirm
the information contained herein with other reliable sources, and are strongly advised to check the product
information sheet provided by the pharmaceutical company for each drug they plan to administer.

9 8 7 6 5 4 3 2 1
Printed in the United States of America
on acid-free paper

CONTENTS

PART TWO
IMPROVING PERFORMANCE OF THE MORAL BRAIN: REMOVING OBSTACLES TO GOOD BEHAVIOR

ACKNOWLEDGMENTS

This book explains a set of new ideas in neuroscience to readers who lack a scientific background. This would have been impossible without the insight, resourcefulness, and organizational skill of Sandra Sherman. I am immensely grateful for all her hard work. She frequently understood the implications of my ideas better than I did, and was able to express them with a clarity that I can only envy. As a former lawyer and English professor now working in finance, Sandra drew connections between my theory and the world outside of my lab, which I think will give this book a far greater resonance.

We both thank our splendid editor at Oxford University Press, Craig Panner, whose generous support we have greatly appreciated. His perspicacious reading benefited our presentation enormously.

I have been thinking about these ideas for a long time. First, I am grateful that the Sarah Lawrence College Library had an excellent comparative religion section, because that is where I got started thinking about the Golden Rule as an ethical universal. Once the main ideas of this book were formulated, I was able to try them out in a course for Neurology residents at Cornell Medical School, in a series of talks organized by the late great Chief of Neurology, Fred

Plum. The lecture received useful criticism from the psychiatrist Marguerite Lederberg, widow of Rockefeller University's President Joshua Lederberg. An abbreviated account of that lecture is in the Springer-Verlag book *Ethical Questions in Brain and Behavior* (1982). *The Altruistic Brain* uses new data, new points of departure, and many new insights from Sandra Sherman to build on my *Neuroscience of Fair Play* (2007) sponsored by the Dana Foundation. Writing from that book is acknowledged here and in the text. Sandra and I also wrote a chapter on Law and Neuroscience in *Current Legal Issues*, Vol. 13 (Oxford University Press, 2010) from which we quote, and we thank Oxford University Press for giving us permission to do so.

Science writer Robin Nixon generously helped me get started with this book. Some of the best aspects of its organization can be credited to her early efforts.

Several scientists gave me excellent leads and advice. Two of my colleagues at the Rockefeller University, neuroscience professors Bruce McEwen and Winrich Freiwald, were outstanding in this regard. Also, my colleague Daniel Kronauer, head of Laboratory of Insect and Social Evolution, provided crucial guidance with regard to my use of terms, enabling me to clarify some of the book's fundamental concepts. Joshua Greene (Harvard University), James Gilligan, M.D. (New York University), Richard Davidson (University of Wisconsin), and Jonathan Haidt (University of Virginia) were also most helpful in contributing to this account of how we are "wired" to behave altruistically. In particular, James Gilligan's positive view of the manuscript, in view of his experience as a psychiatrist overseeing a prison system, has been much appreciated. My administrative assistant at the Rockefeller University, Susan Strider, a professional artist, made all of the illustrations.

Scientists and authors Professor David Barash (University of Washington), Prof. Russell Pearce (Fordham Law School), Prof. Winrich Freiwald (Rockefeller University), and Colin Rule (Stanford) generously took time to read and criticize the text.

Thanks to Mark Greenberg of the Pennsylvania State University who sent us some of his work on helping troubled children. Thanks also to Stephen Post of Stony Brook University Medical Center, who provided us a broad-ranging critique of our ideas, and helped us to contextualize them. Three social workers who know gangs or who have been in a gang, wishing to remain anonymous, looked over the relevant chapters.

Finally, I want to thank Russ Pearce, Mary Gordon, and Colin Rule for sharing with us their own fascinating insights into the operation of moral reciprocity, especially with regard to how it can be applied to make our lives better. Many people are thinking about this issue, and I hope that they will accept *The Altruistic Brain* as a contribution to an ongoing conversation.

INTRODUCTION

Just after New Year's, 2007, New York City—and indeed the world—was transfixed by the heroism of Wesley Autrey, who dove in front of an oncoming subway train to rescue a stranger who had fallen on the tracks. The City awarded Mr. Autrey its highest honor, and Donald Trump publicly wrote him a check. Suddenly, Autrey was everywhere—interviewed, awarded, celebrated—as if everyone wanted to get near him, maybe even inhale a whiff of his magic. "Magic" in this case is not too strong a word, as it quickly became apparent that the source of Mr. Autrey's ability to toss away fear was not readily apparent. How could this guy, standing on a subway platform with his two little daughters, ages four and six, run the risk of death for someone he didn't even know? Autrey's heroism offered the public a chance to think about human motivation where an intended act has no other purpose than pure goodness. It posed questions of enormous complexity, as it made the average person reflect on the limits of his or her own altruistic motivations. A story in the *New York Times* epitomized the dilemma: "Why Our Hero Leapt Onto the Tracks and We Might Not."

The *Times'* story collected the views of several experts: sociologists, psychologists, psychiatrists, an evolutionary biologist, a bioethicist. Each had a theory. Taken together, the story suggested a complicated interplay between Nature and Nurture, starting in Mr. Autrey's brain circuitry but not excluding his training in the Navy. The story's subtext was that no one had all the answers, and that—most likely—there could never be an answer that would suit a one-size-fits-all analysis. Mr. Autrey represented the mosaic of factors that make us human and humane. Depending on the balance of those factors, the story suggested, we might or might not be equipped to follow his example.

Yet what was interesting as a sidebar to all this spirited discussion was Mr. Autrey's own assessment of his behavior. He saw in it nothing unusual, but rather cast his action as a clear-cut, normal act of moral responsibility. The BBC quoted his claim that "I'm still saying I'm not a hero... 'cause I believe all New Yorkers should get into that type of mode." Autrey categorized his act as what anyone should do faced with a similar challenge. "You should do the right thing." Talking with CBS, he made the whole event seem as though it had posed no risk, and that he never calculated the odds of his own survival as he acted to protect others: "I didn't want the man's body to get run over. Plus, I was with my daughters and I didn't want them to see that." As the train approached the man, Autrey's thoughts were entirely practical: "The only thing that popped into my mind was, 'OK, well, go for the gutter [between the tracks]. So I dove in, I pinned him down and once the first car ran over us, my thing with him was to keep him still." Two cars passed over their clinched bodies before the train screeched to a halt but, still concerned about his daughters, Autrey shouted at them from underneath that both men were fine.

Only days later did a certain lovable bravado emerge in Our Hero's demeanor, when he gamely remarked, "Donald Trump's got a check waiting for me. They offered to mail it. I said no, I'd like to meet the Donald, so I can say 'Yo, you're fired.' "

In the following pages, I will suggest that Autrey's low-key acceptance of his own moral courage—his insistence that what he did felt ordinary—provides us a profound insight into the reality of human motivation toward benevolent action. That is, it stands as a key to understanding the various conflicting arguments as to why we act morally, and whether that is what most of us would normally do. There is something of Mr. Autrey in all of us. So I will, in effect, rewrite that *Times* story under the title "Why Our Hero Leapt Onto the Tracks and We Might Too."

The Altruistic Brain offers a transformative intervention in the ongoing discussion of our underlying behavior toward each other and, indeed, it can explain benevolent behaviors in general. I will show how the brain is wired to propel us toward empathic behavior and feelings leading to altruistic behaviors. I will also show how this knowledge of our brain's wiring can, in turn, add to our capacity for benevolence. Though I do not plan to take on the sociologists and psychiatrists, the new scientific theory that follows captures the latest neuroscience research that can be applied to everyday life. It not only can explain why we are good but also help make us better. I am not talking just about heroic altruism, though that is a part of my concern, so much as I am focused on everyday kindness and decency which, when multiplied by billions of such acts in the course of 24 hours, can make each of our days livable. On a broader scale, it makes us inclined to see the goodness in, and hence value our neighbors. Ultimately, it lends power to the sort of group dynamic required for the large-scale actions that modern societies must undertake, and that are necessary to create both a viable sociopolitical regime and, ultimately, a livable planet.

This book advances a new realization of our brain's functions and capacities. In extreme cases, when heroic acts are called for and occur, the type of nerve cell, chemical, and physical mechanisms discussed here explain how those heroic acts can actually occur. *The Altruistic Brain* will thus help us reevaluate our remarkable potential for benevolent action. Though I do not believe that biology is destiny, I will give biology its due, placing neuroscience at the center of a new approach to ethics, one that allows us far greater insight into how we act. If we understand how the brain works, we can design a rational system of ethics having more predictable outcomes, consistent with an actual human nature undistorted by speculation or outmoded ideologies.

OLDER VIEWS

For too long, it has been common wisdom that human nature is essentially selfish. We are taught that our instincts are somehow designed by nature to promote ourselves, and that these "animal" selves must be tamed to fit into "civilization." To a considerable degree, this view reflects Christian doctrine, with most Protestants believing in a type of unforgiving, "total depravity" as the result of Original Sin, and Catholics espousing something similar but with room for a redeeming free will. In *Essential Truths of the Christian Faith* (1992), the noted apologist R.C. Sproul states: "The Bible teaches the total depravity of the human race.... For total depravity means that I and everyone else are depraved or corrupt in the totality of our being. There is no part of us that is left untouched by sin. Our minds, our wills, and our bodies are affected by evil. We speak sinful words, we do sinful deeds, have impure thoughts. Our very bodies suffer from the ravages of sin." According to Christianity, Original Sin is humanity's inheritance, and cannot be expunged. As Sproul puts it, "Perhaps 'radical corruption' is a better term to describe our fallen condition than 'total depravity.' I am using the word 'radical' not so much to mean 'extreme,' but to lean more heavily on its original meaning. 'Radical' comes from the Latin word for 'root' or 'core.' Our problem with sin is that it is rooted in the core of our being. It permeates our hearts."

Indeed, neurobiologists like me have spent lifetimes studying cells in a primitive part of the brain called the hypothalamus, just above the roof of the mouth, and demonstrating how those hypothalamic cells regulate eating, drinking, and even fighting...all behaviors that are essentially "selfish." At the same time, however, evolutionary biologists would affirm that our base instincts have real value for helping individuals and, indeed, our species to survive. Scientists have also done extraordinary work on the origins of sharing and cooperation in early hominids. So what's up? Is it good to be bad? Of course it isn't, though nothing that concerns human nature is ever simple.

Apart from the evolutionary biologists, the average person no doubt would say that there is still a perpetual struggle between good and evil, that is, a 50–50-ness somehow wired into the nature of things. Thus for every 9/11—full of fanaticism, brutality, and hate—there are stories of first responders, willing to give up their lives to pull strangers from the rubble. For those seeking to make progress on defining our capacity to resist temptation, false ideology, and greed, the question is: where do we find the raw materials that make up a more benign version of human nature?

It turns out these raw materials are in our brains. The human brain is actually programmed to make us care for others. Many of our basic drives, reactions, and skills are more products of nature than of nurture. The innate biology of the human brain compels us to be kind. That is, we are *wired* for goodwill.

When we seek clarity about human goodness, the real question comes down not so much to philosophy—which is at a level of abstraction always permitting exceptions, caveats, and indeed circularity—but empiricism, measuring the real-world experience of actual humans as they behave toward one another. In this context, the word "goodness" has lately become associated with notions of empathy, a hugely variant concept that generally means the capacity to perceive and share feelings as experienced by others. Note the term "as," because empathy has come to be valued as a present-tense, real-time reaction to another's physical and emotional state. The noted primatologist Frans De Waal suggests that its most important characteristic is the capacity to "be affected by and share the emotional state of another." Nancy Eisenberg goes further, pointing to a certain mimetic quality, "an affective response that stems from the apprehension or comprehension of another's emotional state or condition, and that is similar to what the other person is feeling or would be expected to feel."

Empathy is not simply a generalized benevolence, which perhaps we might expect from Plato's enlightened Philosopher King, but a specific response to another person (or group) engendered by a defined, immediate situation. In other words, empathy requires an emotional and cognitive connection. Scientists have sought to measure empathy at various levels—behavioral, to be sure, but also physiological (as in facial or other nonverbal expressions). Such measurements have given rise to the famous notion of "emotional contagion," as registered in the person who does the empathizing. At such levels, however, benevolence can seem attenuated, as much a fact of the laboratory as it is of human relations. In *The Altruistic Brain*, I examine the unmediated response of one human being to another, a potential that is wired into everybody's brain.

While philosophy, biology, and psychology have pondered the social side of human nature more or less forever, over the last few decades neuroscience has taken a brave new step toward finally addressing who we are in context with other human beings. How do we get along? What makes us like or dislike each other? Why do we cooperate? These are controversial subjects for any science to tackle, which is why neuroscientists have only begun to broach them now, when our techniques are maturing and we have a better grip on understanding the human mind.

Indeed, some philosophers such as Patricia Churchland seek to integrate neuroscience into a theory of moral behavior. Her most famous study, *Braintrust*, explores what she describes as "neuroethics," the neurobiological basis of consciousness, the self, and free will. Yet this and similar studies, though illuminating, do not formulate a nitty-gritty theory or morality based on nerve cell biology. They are at a level of generality that is more speculative, more recognizably "philosophical" than a specifically scientific study would ever be. *The Altruistic Brain*, therefore, reverses this approach. It uses hard science—that is, hard neuroscience—to propose a detailed theory of moral conduct founded exclusively on what we know about brain function.

NEUROSCIENCE PROGRESSING

Indeed, neuroscience is the only science possessing the capacity to explain exactly how or why humans can regularly behave in a good and ethical way. None of the other sciences—let alone social sciences—possesses the tools. Neuroscience starts from the premise that all of our social behaviors are products of the human mind, and that the brain is the organ of the mind. Thus to be serious about ethical behavior, we need access to the best contemporary work on brain mechanisms for behavior.

Unfortunately, neuroscience research during the past 100 years or so has emphasized beginning with very simple problems such as behaviors in lower animals, spinal reflexes, or elementary motivations such as hunger. Many of the smartest people in this field still avoid facing questions of complexity. Indeed, the choice to work on manageable problems characterized most of my own career, as my lab addressed problems involving steroid hormone effects on simple brains and behaviors.

I therefore propose the Altruistic Brain Theory (ABT), which represents a leap, both for me personally and for neuroscience, to consider how the brain actually produces altruistic behavior. In one sense, I have been thinking about the neuromechanics of altruism for years, slowly piecing together literally hundreds of studies; it has been part of my mental calisthenics for years. But in another sense, actually proposing this theory—that is, explaining in detail how we are wired to be good—is a brand new departure. It is like going from zero to 60 mph, or maybe 90, all at once on a different track. While some of my colleagues have just begun to broach the subject, they haven't dared accelerate toward anything as complete or as comprehensive as ABT. Why? It is safer to get grants for topics where they show results. Our knowledge of crucial structures and functions in the brain is rapidly developing, so why can't there be a mechanism for altruism that neuroscience can describe? Thus ABT represents a kind of perfect storm of audacity, awareness, and insight. We are accustomed to this kind of storm in, say, the humanities, when suddenly there is Modernism or the French New Wave. Well, that same kind of sudden actualization can happen in science as well. It happens because a whole lot of data can be "out there," until finally it all comes together at once.

The emergence of ABT all at once may take some getting used to, as it may have immense social implications. It is not like other scientific developments that, though important to scientists, do not speak directly to society at large. In this latter category I am thinking, for example, of the discovery of the Higgs boson or, on a much less cosmic level, the production of mice with knockout genes. Even if the entire field of particle physics is revolutionized by the discover of the Higgs boson, how is that going to affect how we live our lives? To ask that question is to answer it. But if suddenly a neuroscientist demonstrates that, almost certainly, the human race is predisposed toward benevolence, then isn't there an immediate connection between science and "real life?" The reason that I was willing to go for broke on ABT, and get out of my comfort zone into something genuinely big, was that I wanted to make that connection emphatically. I didn't want to write another book that was just for scientists. I wanted to write something that could help change how real people organize their lives. I wanted to connect with readers directly about a subject in which, as it turns out, science has a lot of new insight.

Of course, an important part of making that connection will be to convey to you some sense of my own discovery. A new "theory" is not something tangible—like a new kind of laboratory mouse—that you can hold in your hand and inspect. It is an abstraction, an idea. So how can I prove to you that it exists, that it has a reality that is (1) based on measurable, tangible data and (2) explains phenomena that you can see (every good scientific idea *explains* things). Well, in terms of showing you the data that I relied on, I will take you on a discovery into labs around the world. I will introduce you to the scientists doing the experiments and writing the papers on which ABT is based. In terms of showing you how the theory actually works to explain human behavior, I will break down both ordinary and world-class events into the neurohormonal steps that brought that behavior about. That is, I will show you what happened in the brain to make an off-duty fireman put down his golf clubs, race into Manhattan, and give up his life to save victims on 9/11. Thus while ABT is abstract, it is also dramatic in terms of how I discovered it and how it operates in real life. I invite you to follow me.

ALTRUISTIC BRAIN THEORY

As I show in the following pages, good behavior in humans can be explained much more straightforwardly than previously understood. The human brain processes altruism in five specific steps:

> Step 1: Your central nervous system registers the act that you are about to perform toward another person. A vast amount of data, gathered during electrical recordings from nerve cells of experimental subjects, proves that the brain signals a movement to itself before the movement occurs.

Step 2: You picture the person who will be the target of this act. This step in the theory is necessary for the later evaluation of the act toward that person.

Step 3: The image of that person blurs with that of one's self. This step is crucial, as it provides the basis for treating the other person like oneself. It is also an easy step to accomplish because it does not require greater precision of performance by the nervous system but, instead, less precise performance.

Step 4: You experience "feeling," which allows you to evaluate the consequences of the potential act. Once the act is represented in your brain and your combined self/other image is in place, neurons in your prefrontal cortex place a positive or a negative value on the act. The Altruistic Brain has been activated.

Step 5: You decide whether or not to act. According to Step 4, if the consequence of the act is good, you perform it. If it is bad, you don't.

Each step takes place below the level of consciousness and is completed within the tiniest fraction of a second. Because the brain makes a quick, split-second decision to act morally, I call the mechanism for it the Altruistic Brain, and thus the theory for how this mechanism operates is the ABT.

After centuries of debate over whether humanity is fundamentally flawed (as blamed on Eve) or particularly benevolent (as proposed by the philosopher David Hume), neuroscience is ready to provide the answer: We are good. In fact, the guiding principle of a healthy human brain is "First act morally, then ask why."

That is, we are instinctively good, and the idea is now ready for prime time. Thus though I have included some uncompromising brain science, *The Altruistic Brain* is intended as a practical book, pointing the way toward how science can enhance our social relations. Some chapters in the second half of the book offer real-life applications of ABT. They suggest that if we can accept that people are basically good, then we should institutionalize this concept in order to promote trust. *Trust is of enormous practical utility.* For example, if parties to what is known as a "dispute resolution proceeding" (a less formal alternative to a full-blown trial) are encouraged to appreciate each other's capacity to empathize, then they are more likely to achieve levels of trust necessary to produce a settlement. Trust-building is crucial to all sorts of relationships, whether in negotiations across a table or in resolving online disputes on eBay or similar e-commerce websites. (The Better Business Bureau motto is "Start With Trust"). Trust is crucial to divorce proceedings, where people cannot even stand each other but can still trust in each other's reasonable desire to work through the issues. I will argue that because empathy is a key motivator of trust, ABT could be recognized as a useful view of who people are at the earliest stages of seemingly intractable negotiations, giving people added incentive to rely on trust, and not to shut their minds down even before beginning to talk.

My concept of an Altruistic Brain did not originate from any single, particular discovery in my own lab. Rather, several years ago, I read philosophy and religion extensively, and realized with a growing excitement that religious and philosophical demands for reciprocally benevolent behavior appeared to be remarkably consistent across all of these writings.

As I read, it occurred to me that the universal nature of dictates for human benevolence—Golden Rule–like requirements across centuries and continents—indicated a basis in biology. I concluded that I should start to think about whether the brain, the organ on which I have now worked for more than 50 years, played a role in shaping this apparently universal inclination.

While my research had heretofore dealt with mechanisms for simple instinctive behaviors, it suddenly flashed into my mind that I could (with much more thinking!) formulate a detailed brain mechanism to explain how human beings behave well toward each other.

The Altruistic Brain will put my findings in context with the most recent developments across the field of neuroscience. I examine the results of scientific tools, such as brain images produced by functional magnetic resonance imagery (fMRI), and apply them to a physical/cellular analysis of how we behave well toward each other. I also present the overwhelming statistical, psychological, evolutionary, genetic, and neurological evidence that the human brain is wired for goodwill, which propels us toward empathic displays of altruism, like Wesley Autrey's leap onto the subway tracks.

I also examine the unmediated response of one human being to another, a potential that is wired into everybody's brain. I present these brain mechanisms with the knowledge of a working neuroscientist who has been studying how the brain regulates behavior—normal and abnormal—for his entire career. Just as MIT linguist Noam Chomsky speculated that our brains are wired to produce grammatical sentences, so I demonstrate (using Chomsky as a useful analogy) that our brains are wired to produce altruistic behavior. I offer real-life nerve cell examples of how this behavior occurs, which helps explain who we are with respect to our behaviors toward other individuals—our ethical, moral behaviors, or in some cases a lack thereof.

Note that last phrase, "lack thereof." Even as my research explains the neurological mechanisms that foster ethical behaviors, it also acknowledges shortcomings in the behaviors of both individuals and groups that often lead to violent impulses. Once we understand these impulses, however, we can seek to allay them and allow the Altruistic Brain to proceed uninterrupted. I discuss how we can create circumstances that will help rectify the balance between pro- and antisocial behaviors. In this regard, several chapters offer contributions toward a practical ethics aimed at elevating individuals' social behavior. If we know with certainty that we can tap into our own and others' altruistic capacities, then we can work (as individuals and in groups) toward removing obstacles in the way of giving effect to those capacities.

In extreme cases, when heroic acts are called for and occur, the brain mechanisms—nerve cells' and neural circuits' chemical and physical mechanisms—explain how those heroic acts can actually occur. *The Altruistic Brain* will thus help us reevaluate our remarkable potential for benevolent action. Though I do not believe that biology is destiny, I will give biology its due, placing neuroscience at the center of a new approach to ethics, one that allows us far greater insight into how we act. If we understand how the brain works, we can design an ethics having more predictable outcomes, consistent with an actual human nature undistorted by speculation or outmoded ideologies.

WHAT IS A SCIENTIFIC THEORY?

Having sketched the five steps of ABT, I want to make clear what a scientific "theory" actually is. Evolution is a theory. So is Relativity. So is Plate Tectonics. That is, a theory in science is not just a glorified hunch, but rather a deep and systematic explanation of some aspect of the natural world based on a substantial body of facts that scientists have repeatedly observed and confirmed. Such theories aim to predict and explain. *Scientific* theories are grounded in years of rigorous research—not just by one researcher, but by a whole community of scientists working on ideas that contribute to the theory.

When you read about the Altruistic Brain "theory," therefore, you are reading about an explanation developed by means of the scientific method. In this regard, *The Altruistic Brain* is a little like a work of theoretical physics, in which a scientist faces a large body of facts, thinks about them, talks with other scientists about them, thinks some more, comes to a realization similar to the last steps of solving a Rubik's Cube...and then writes up the result of this process for the wider world. In the theory, almost everything finally falls into place. In theoretical physics, the result might be, say, string theory. In the case of this book, the result is to explain a form of higher human behavior without supposing any extraordinary or supernatural capacities of the human brain.

Because science is such a communal enterprise, all the research explained in *The Altruistic Brain* did not—and could not have—come entirely from my lab. Nor was it all dedicated to locating the sources of altruism in humans. The research concerned dozens, maybe hundreds, of insights that, when pieced together, led me to conclude that an Altruistic Brain mechanism existed. This is how science operates. No one person "discovers" a theory. Nor does he or she necessarily make all the requisite findings in his or her own lab. Rather, science inches along collectively, often hitting a number of points until they all more or less fit together. Where there is a lot "more" than "less," we have a viable theory.

As every scientist knows, science does not just wrap up a theory in a nice neat package. Though ABT is actually a lot neater than most, it is, as I said, like a Rubik's Cube, proposed by me only after lots of moves by me and other people. There may still be holes in this theory, which hopefully time and further research will address. ABT aims at the future, and at how we will finally understand our own motivations. It aims at a point in time when we will acknowledge that no "God gene" or Higher Power is required to motivate us to be good.

In the chapters that follow, I describe many of the moves that finally led me to piece together pieces of the puzzle. While the moves, joyfully, came from many of my friends and colleagues, I put them together in a way that begins to describe a plausible approach to a complex question

We have developed collective preconceptions about each other that ABT challenges, and over time can help to dispel. If we could more easily accept each other's inherent decency (i.e., if our institutions modeled such an approach), we might be better equipped to cooperate and, ultimately, develop a kind of practical trust. This could provide a useful means toward healing and toward enabling people to succeed at relationship formation. "Trust" is a form of empathy, of seeing something of oneself in another such that we can *reasonably anticipate* that our words and feelings will be understood. In trying to map the coordinates of trust onto neuroanatomy, *The Altruistic Brain* is ultimately an exercise in how to make the possible feasible; it starts from what we are capable of and points the way, through our own understanding of those capabilities, to how we can better exist together. It tries to answer the question: "If we can now, for the first time, really accept that we are inclined toward reciprocal morality, how can we put that knowledge to use in everyday life?"

In fact, everyday life is the key. In June, 2012, the *New York Times* ran a story about parents' monitoring their children's online activity. Several readers wrote letters in response, but one got right to the heart of the issue, observing that "As a mother of four teenagers, I have found it best to trust that the lessons of respect for others, being a good neighbor and being held accountable for your own actions will extend into their electronic world and guide their behavior." She added—in an insight that might be a snapshot of this book—that "Trust and open communication seem like far more powerful tools than electronic snooping." Clearly, this parent has faith in her children's essential decency, in part because she is doing all that she can to preserve and promote it. This book is intended to encourage us all to apply such lessons.

I am inspired to take this route by Paul Romer's notion of meta-ideas, which he defines as "ideas that help us get better at discovering ideas," or "ideas about how to support the production and transmission of other ideas." Romer, a professor at Stanford Business School, focuses on how certain social formations—libraries, the patent system, research universities—are actually *ideas* that create conditions for enhanced creativity. They make possible exchanges between people that lead to whole new concepts: transistors, for example, which came out of the ferment at Bell Labs. Accepting the notion that humans are wired for benevolence is just such a meta-idea, in that, as I will suggest, it leads to an array of new approaches to how we might organize both our personal and large-scale social relations.

Of course, I must acknowledge that, for some readers, I will be sailing right into the headwinds of their tremendous skepticism. From their perspective, we are all egoists, doing good only when it serves our purposes. Professor Judith Lichtenberg of Georgetown University recently articulated this point: "One reason people deny that altruism exists is that, looking inward, they doubt the purity of their own motives. We know that even when we appear to act unselfishly, other reasons for our behavior often rear their heads: the prospect of a future favor, the boost to reputation, or simply the good feeling that comes from appearing to act unselfishly. As Kant and Freud observed, people's true motives may be hidden, even (or perhaps especially) from themselves."

Well, I will argue that while in some theoretical number of cases altruism may be only apparent—the product of craft and calculation—back in the real world of brain circuitry, our altruistic response to another's need is our default response. That is, altruistic acts are, in fact, what they seem to be: acts that are inherently good with no ulterior motive. This is because they are *natural*. We may doubt our own motives out of a certain admirable humility, or on the assumption that as complex humans we could never act out of "simple" kindness. But if at times we still have other motives for doing good, then so what? Our brains are wired to propel us in that direction in any case, irrespective of any auxiliary calculations. For those who are skeptical about human kindness, the objective of *The Altruistic Brain* is to change your mind about how the mind works. None of this is mysterious. But seeing how our brains naturally produce altruistic behaviors seems to me to be the most exciting and optimistic subject that I could be writing about, given current scientific knowledge.

So in closing, I'd like to riff on an idea in the latest book by Nobel laureate Eric Kandel, *The Age of Insight: The Quest to Understand the Unconscious in Art, Mind, and Brain, from Vienna 1900 to the Present* (Random House, 2012). In examining how neuroscience can illuminate our understanding of art, Kandel responds to critics who think that "scientific" analysis of artistic production—where such production rests on capacities of immense human complexity—can offer only a diminished idea of how we actually react to art:

> Science seeks to understand complex processes by reducing them to their essential actions and studying the interplay of those actions—and this reductionist approach extends to art as well.... Some people are concerned that reductionist analysis will diminish our fascination with art, that it will trivialize art and deprive it of its special force, thereby reducing the beholder's share to an ordinary brain function. I argue to the contrary, that by encouraging a dialogue between science and art and by encouraging a focus on one mental process at a time, reductionism can expand our vision and give us new insights into the nature and creation of art. These new insights will enable us to perceive unexpected aspects of art that derive from the relationships between biological and psychological phenomena.

If we were to substitute the term "empathy" or "altruism" in this paragraph for "art," Kandel's argument could just as well apply to what I seek to accomplish in *The Altruistic Brain*. That is, far from trivializing empathy and kindness, and reducing our concept of these capabilities to the level of "ordinary brain function," I want to show how adding a scientific valence to the study of our best nature will increase our fascination with how we attained that nature. I want to show how complex human societies could not have evolved but for the brain's extraordinary wiring that favors benevolence. Kandel's argument is that when it comes to brain function, scientific reductionism is ultimately the best way to appreciate the brain's complexity. I hope that you will ultimately agree.

PART I

EVIDENCE FOR ALTRUISTIC BRAIN THEORY

[1]

THE BIOLOGICAL/
EVOLUTIONARY ROOTS OF
ALTRUISM

When approaching reciprocally altruistic behaviors from a biological perspective, scientists have followed two paths. One explains the cellular and physical steps involved in producing empathetic behaviors. This is my approach in the Altruistic Brain Theory (ABT). The other path to understanding such behavior, currently very popular, has aspects of *Indiana Jones*: biologists brave the jungle to observe animal behavior, emerging with evolutionary scenarios depicting how animals—especially primates such as monkeys and chimpanzees—got to behave in a seemingly empathic way. Of course, these adventurers leave out a crucial step: evolutionary development must, in fact, *still* work through brain mechanisms. But because we only recently acquired the detailed knowledge based on brain research that makes such jungle forays seem less than ideal, the animal-based, evolutionary approach has provided a serviceable explanation.

Indeed, this chapter argues that understanding this "heroic" approach to altruism can help us appreciate the concept from a scientific perspective, providing a good precursor for a neuroscientific analysis. Before getting to brain mechanisms, therefore, let's discuss these evolutionary ideas. These ideas, originally intended to explain how the brain's mechanisms for altruism came about, also support claims that we can describe mechanisms for how these behaviors *operate*. That is, evolutionary theories for altruistic behavior also stimulate scientific thinking about how such behavior works.

For background, let's begin with some basic concepts in evolutionary biology. The late Rockefeller University population geneticist Theodosius Dobzhansky observed that "Nothing in biology makes sense except in the light of evolution." If we accept this view, as I do, then the idea would be to determine how it bears on altruism and, indeed, moral reciprocity. Following Dobzhansky, other scientists note that humans are by "nature great cooperators." Well then, how is the puzzle of altruism explained? What exactly are the evolutionary mechanisms that produce reciprocally empathic behaviors?

To introduce this evolutionary thinking, I try to imagine a scene from our evolutionary past. Thousands of years ago, anthropologists tell us, the basis for empathic social interaction was already there. Where did it come from? Scientists have defined a new dividing line between humans and other animals, such that a "human" will possess our hyper-developed social skills. These skills include language, of course, but perhaps more importantly our ability to "read" others' minds. That is, we understand from someone's posture, tone, or facial expression what that person is feeling and/or what he or she may desire. For example, a human toddler readily perceives that an adult with full hands staring at a closed door wants to go through that door but needs help, so the toddler will try to lend the adult a hand. A monkey is unlikely to offer a paw, even to another monkey—not out of callousness but out of ignorance.

How did such helping behavior develop? How did we become wired for such willing displays of beneficent behavior? Evolutionary biologists grappling with the evolution of human social behavior have tended to favor any one of three theoretical answers to how human social behaviors have gradually developed. Unfortunately, however, they treat such theories as though each were mutually exclusive of the others—indeed, competing in a tournament, so that if one were important, the others could not be. Such biologists argue with each other in the media, often assigning confusing, disparate terms to explain (and justify) their separate, uncompromising approaches.

Yes, the evolution of social behavior is a crucially important topic, but I disagree with theorists who treat the field as a zero-sum game, limited to one or another specific theory of kinship-based altruism. Instead of taking this conventional approach, I treat three different theories in a manner in which they could all operate at the same time, pulling in the same direction in a manner that will explain the evolution of human behavior toward the altruism explained by ABT.

Viewing the field of evolutionary biology from the outside, it seems apparent that evolutionary theorists argue over which of the three mechanisms—"selfish DNA," or "kin selection," or "group selection"—is *the* most important. But as a neuroscientist, I can see how the three could work together to produce altruistic behaviors. As another outsider to the field, Ken Binmore, economics professor at University College London states, reciprocally altruistic acts serve the purpose of "ensuring" each of the individuals against bad stuff; in this regard, he makes no distinctions between various evolutionary approaches. The same (if various) theories that address how food sharing by lower animals has evolved can also be called on to address how sophisticated cooperative behaviors among modern humans have developed over time.

THREE EVOLUTIONARY THEORIES ABOUT THE DEVELOPMENT OF ALTRUISM

1. Selfish DNA

Picture each organism saying "Since I have selfish DNA, I behave with a narrowly defined self-interest to make sure that my own DNA is passed on to the next generation." This will obviously work to explain some forms of social behavior, but now we must delve into the field of evolutionary biology to see how it would help explain the development of altruistic, prosocial behavior.

Early in the last century, the British statistician Ronald A. Fisher turned his attention to natural variations in traits among individuals in large populations. According to Oren Harman in *The Price of Altruism*, Fisher thought about how to integrate genetics into the explanation of variations among individuals. Harman observes that "the centerpiece" of Fisher's book was "the fundamental theorem of natural selection" among individuals, to determine who would live long enough to reproduce: "The rate of increase of fitness of any organism is equal to its *genetic* variance in fitness at that time" (italics mine). Applying this genetic approach to the analysis of social behaviors among animals and humans, the British biologist Richard Dawkins wrote in *The Selfish Gene* that insofar as the selfish gene influences behavior, it would regulate behavior in such a way as to increase its frequency in the gene pool. That goal simply requires that the individual whose behavior is affected by that gene should survive as long as possible and reproduce as frequently as possible.

In fact, some genes are so selfish that they induce conflicts within the genome itself. So-called "selfish genetic elements" are defined by the theoretical biologist John Werren as having "characteristics enhancing their own transmission relative to the rest of the individual genome, but neutral or detrimental to the organism as a whole." In these cases, an individual gene containing a DNA sequence that makes that gene really active, sending many of its cellular signals, upsets the optimal balance among genes. A different kind of genomic conflict emerges when you consider the copy of each gene that comes from the mother as opposed to the copy of that same gene from the father. In this case, the "conflict" within the genome itself is between the copy on the chromosome that originated in the mother versus the copy on the chromosome that came from the father. Which copy dominates and is expressed—the father's or the mother's—can affect biologically important behaviors.

Though the bulk of his book emphasizes self-centered behavior (one chapter is entitled "You Scratch My Back, I'll Ride on Yours"), Dawkins is willing to soften his hard-nosed approach to social behavior when talking about humans. In the case of humans, he thinks we should consider the cultural transmission of influences on behavior. In any culture, an individual may imitate the behavior of another person, usually older and admired. Is it possible, then, to think of a "unit of cultural transmission" analogous to a gene? Dawkins, citing the word "imitate," comes up with "mimeme" and then the more euphonious word "meme" to represent this unit. This additional form of behavioral regulation inherently opens up new possibilities for explaining cultural forms that are specifically human and not selfish. Dawkins gives as examples "religion, music and ritual dancing." Under some circumstances, the contingencies of cultural reward might even prevent us from behaving selfishly. Instead, as Dawkins is willing to consider in one chapter, "Nice Guys (Can) Finish First." The importance of this view is that Dawkins deduces that we have the power to defy the selfish genes of our birth. Thus strong and civilized cultural support can overcome an unfortunate genetic heritage. It is important for us that strong cultural support for prosocial behavior may prevent social problems that could otherwise emerge from individuals who, for example, possess over-aggressive tendencies.

2. Kin Selection Theory

"I help this person because he is related to me and if he survives through the age of reproduction, parts of my DNA will be passed on. The closer he is related, the more of my DNA he has."

As E. O. Wilson explains in *The Superorganism*, kin selection theory arose in 1932, when the British biologist J. B. S. Haldane wrote that "A consideration of these (altruistic) traits involves the consideration of small groups. For a character of this type can only spread through the population if the genes determining it are borne by a group of related individuals whose chances of leaving offspring are increased by the presence of these genes…" That is, an individual's behavior will benefit his relatives even if that behavior might not be great for his own sake.

Kin Selection Theory sat around for decades until William D. Hamilton refurbished it mathematically in 1964, renaming it "inclusive fitness." Hamilton, born on an island in the Nile and educated at Cambridge, was a biologist who, according to Oren Harman, "inherited his father's aptitude for math." He wanted to follow Ronald Fisher so as to achieve a quantitative explanation of altruistic behavior—which he did. His equation told us that if you multiply the benefit of your potential altruistic act times the closeness of your relation to the beneficiary of that act, and if that multiplication product exceeds the cost (to you) of your act, then you will perform that altruistic act.

But Hamilton was just the start. Harvard's mathematical biologist Martin Nowak most admires how Robert Trivers presents kin selection. In a 1971 paper in the *Quarterly Review of Biology*, Trivers coined the term "reciprocal altruism"—not just "an unselfish concern for the welfare of others," but a pattern of social behavior shared with another individual through a large number of repetitions in a long-lived community. When applied to people who are related to each other, as in kin selection, reciprocal altruism "appeals to common sense," in Nowak's words. After all, if you are about to do something that will save your brother's life, because your brother is highly likely to share many of your same genes, your altruistic act effectively increases the chance of passing on your genes to the next generation. Importantly, for the same reason, your brother would do the same for you.

So from a purely genetic perspective, kin selection works effectively to share in the explanation of altruistic behaviors, and emotionally it makes sense. However, some biologists have thought that it is too restrictive. Hence there is a third theory, group selection.

3. Group Selection Theory

"I help this person because he is part of the same group that I belong to. If the group survives, in general, then both my kin and I can pass on our DNA to the next generation."

Many biologists realized that we don't have to be related to those toward whom we are altruistic. Virtually all of the examples in this chapter attest to this idea. Therefore, we need a broader, less restrictive principle to account for this altruistic social behavior. Group selection provides the breadth; at the same time, it is recognized as the weakest, slowest way to increase the level of altruism in an evolving society (Figure 1.1).

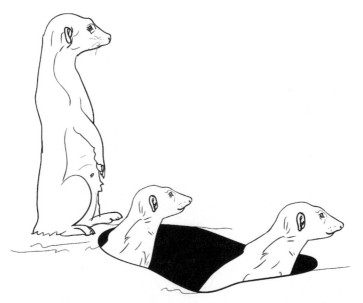

Figure 1.1 To warn other members of their colony, prairie dogs will expose themselves to danger by standing at one of their burrow entrances to watch for predators.

Put another way, group selection gives us a way to talk about how cultural influences could foster altruistic acts. Culture counts, but it does not provide the genetic hammer that (1) "selfish DNA" and (2) "kin selection" provide. But as Edward O. Wilson emphasizes in his recent book, *The Social Conquest of Earth*, it works. Aside from all the casual, real-life examples that we could bring to bear, consider Elizabeth Dunn's work concerning the emotional consequences of spending money on others under controlled laboratory circumstances. She knew the psychological literature describing how people enjoy helping acquaintances and donating to charity. So she used a large sample of more than 600 Americans to look for the emotional effect of "investing income in others rather than oneself." Comparing subjects' different ways of spending money on a monthly basis—rent, food, other expenses—she found that their general happiness was not related to spending on themselves, but correlated much more closely with what they spent on gifts for others and donations to charity. In a smaller sample of individuals who benefited from unexpected economic windfalls, the only measure that predicted those people's happiness was what the authors called "prosocial spending": again, buying something for someone else or donating to charity.

The anthropologist Joan Silk has also studied the remarkable degree of altruism among humans. In her words, "food sharing and division of labor play an important role in all human societies and cooperation extends beyond the bounds of close kinship and networks of reciprocating partners." Silk writes that across a range of nonhuman primate species, "social bonds seem to enhance the ability to cope with chronic stressors, such a slow social status, or acute stressors, such as the loss of preferred partners...." Primatologist Dorothy Cheney pushes the argument further. In some cases, she writes, "some animals may recognize other individual's *intentions*..." (italics mine), thus permitting an even higher degree of cooperation. Cheney and her husband, Robert Seyfarth, write in their paper, "The evolutionary origins of friendship," that "natural selection therefore appears to have favored individuals who are motivated to form long-term bonds per se, not just bonds with kin." Social bonds count, and maintaining them by means of kind, giving behaviors toward others in your group is prevalent among humans, as well as among nonhumans such as chimpanzees and baboons.

But let's back up a little. From a hard-boiled, mathematical point of view, does group selection make sense? Martin Nowak believes that within a group, "cooperation can emerge out of nothing more than the rational calculation of self-interest." Ever the mathematician, Nowak further claims that "group selection allows the evolution of cooperation provided that one thing holds good: the ratio of the benefits to cost exceeds the value of one plus the ratio of group size to the number of groups. Thus group selection works well if there are many small groups and not so well if there are a few large lumbering groups." Nowak's calculations indicate that, as mentioned, group selection may provide a relatively weak and slow way to explain the evolution of cooperative and ethical behaviors. Yet there is no reason that group selective mechanisms could not *add to or even multiply* the beneficial effects of kin selection and the operation of "selfish DNA." Moreover, group selection becomes stronger when individuals know that there will be repeated interactions with one another.

THREE EVOLUTIONARY ROUTES WORKING TOGETHER

Viewing the field from the perspective of a neuroscientist it appears, as mentioned, that while evolutionary biologists argue over the best path to cooperative behavior, in fact all three explanations for the evolution of altruism can augment each other. All three levels of evolutionary theory could be operating at the same time. Selfish DNA, level 1, is most ruthlessly efficient, but is also the narrowest. Group selection, level 3, is broadest, though the least direct and likely the slowest to benefit. Not only can the three add to each other, but the relative importance of each also will vary according to time period and the culture in question. Collectively, however, and no matter how the importance of each varies over time, the convergence of all three evolutionary paths ultimately points toward the development of brain mechanisms favoring altruism. It does not matter which of these paths was more important—a fact that in any case we cannot measure—so much as it *does* matter that they all support the notion that evolution allowed the brain to develop in ways that support benevolent behavior.

But how did altruism start? As a neuroscientist, I cannot give you as long and will not give you as polemical an answer as a field biologist who is out in the field with nonhuman primates. I will, however, spotlight some ideas concerning origins that will provide background to the next chapter on the neuroanatomy of altruism. These include (1) better hunting and (2) better care for the young; the third idea, machine-based cooperation, will directly lead into my discussion of brain mechanisms.

Better hunting. It seems obvious that a group of hunters in which everyone cooperates could do better than an individual hunting alone. I note that altruism—leading to reciprocal altruism and indeed to a history and expectation of reciprocal altruism—is fundamental to trust, and to the kinds of cooperation involved in successful hunting. Thus many evolutionary biologists have suggested that the driving force for the first significant and long-lasting acts of cooperation was the ability to hunt better game. This theory says that while individual hominids could kill small game, such as a hare, they needed to work together to kill bigger game, such as a stag. Afterwards, there was no point in trying to steal all the meat for oneself or to "defect after cooperating," as the game theorists would put it, because there was too much to eat alone. And because we evolved long before refrigeration was invented, prey would just rot in the hot African sun (or be stolen by other carnivores) before breakfast. So Nature determined that we learn to share.

Better care for the young. How the need for optimal care of the young contributed to the development of generalized altruistic tendencies is a more complicated notion than the better-hunting scenario. Ideas about how such cooperation started involve back-and-forth interactions with children, the presence of other helpful women, as well as the father who might have different interests—a scene of interactions far more subtle than catching a wild boar. The theory here is that selection pressures resulted in choosing more cooperative, empathetic individuals because it is so hard to raise adaptive, highly intelligent children to the point that they themselves can reproduce. One of the reasons children must be born in a state of relative helplessness is the problem of getting the baby out of the womb. We may never know the exact reason, but the average human brain size increased dramatically to about twice the size of other primate brains roughly 2 million years ago. In the process, babies' heads became too big to pass through the narrow birth canal of the bipedal human ancestor. Nature's solution was to get the babies out sooner, before their big heads made exiting impossible. As a result, all human babies are born "prematurely" in comparison to our closest ape relatives. Once freed from the restrictions of the birth canal, the brain grows rapidly. The brain almost doubles in size in the first year; the rate slows somewhat only in the second year of life. Still, human babies remain comparatively helpless. This lack of initial ability to survive on their own will be associated with developmental potential that, in the long run, confers an advantage, but that poses an immediate problem for mothers and others nearby. All these facts contribute to the need, as mentioned, for better care for the young.

A Little Help, Please

Now, mothers have predominantly been selected for kindness, caring-concern, and empathy. As De Waal puts it, "Mammalian females with care-giving tendencies have out-reproduced those without for 180 million years." But as primatologist Sarah Hrdy explains in her book, *Mothers and Others*, over the course of evolutionary history, "at some point human mothers began to bear offspring *too costly* to rear by themselves" (emphasis mine). That is, the time and metabolic energy required by offspring forced evolutionary changes in our species that resulted in mothers getting help. Hrdy reasons that this made a mother's commitment to any given child contingent on her perception of social support, her confidence that other women would chip in and help her raise that child. Young and inexperienced mothers, without confidence of that support, may, in fact, abandon a child. Hrdy's key point is that the need for support when raising young had the likely effect of contributing to the social and, perhaps especially, the sexual selection pressures that helped us develop neural circuits of goodwill. With the needs of cooperative breeders, displays of altruism likely became potent aphrodisiacs, with everyone competing to show their goodness. Evolutionary-minded psychiatrist Randolph Nesse, an opinion leader in the field of primatology, suggests that in this manner sexual selection likely "promoted the capacity for altruism in a runaway intensification," thus causing humans to develop and exhibit progressively greater capacities for kindness.

In childrearing, sensitivity to others definitely works both ways: it is no accident that the first skills that babies develop are social. They are, from day one, sensitive to faces, touch, and voices. They are greatly in tune with their caregivers' mood. Before they learn to use their hands or legs, they learn to smile. Their cries change from automatic impulses to actual communications of displeasure. Talking and walking develop literally in step with one another, as if nature hasn't yet decided which is most important for survival. Interestingly, by the time locomotion is fully in place, the parent–infant bond is considered sealed, guaranteeing extra protection as dangers mount.

Hrdy explains that "Humans, who of all the apes produce the largest, slowest-maturing, and most costly babies, also breed the fastest." And the pressures of natural selection toward better infant care would have continued after babyhood, as the needs for human adult care are longer than for any other animal. These pressures lead to a phenomenon called "alloparenting." That is, from a human evolutionary perspective, mothers are only part of the story. While secure attachment to the mother is primary, having other attachments is critical for building perspective-taking abilities and other skills of intelligence. Studies across cultures have shown that children do best when they have at least three relationships that—from different angles and locations—consistently send the message, "Hey, I understand and care about you." These relations are to the mother, other women, and the father.

Field studies of primates, as well as cross-cultural studies of humans, show that the more help a mother has the more babies she can have, and the more likely her offspring are to survive. With extra hands available, she weans each baby more quickly than she would otherwise, and thus is likely to become fertile again sooner. Moreover, the mother's social status as a popular, altruistic female also helps more of her children survive until adulthood.

Mothers with the social skills to attract alloparents—family members and fathers who actually possess willingness to help—would have continued to pass more of their genes into the next generation. Fittingly, the genes governing human behavior, that is, those involved with the brain and other parts of the central nervous system, are thought by some to be among the fastest evolving in the human genome. That is, the more babies who have sprung from socially skilled mothers (and socially skilled extended families) the more babies who will themselves have babies who have their parents' social skills and, perhaps, their neuronal and hormonal makeup. Hence their greater popularity, love, and companionship will drive human evolution toward ever increasing levels of social prowess. As historian of the family Stephanie Coontz observed in 1992, "Children do best in societies where childrearing is considered too important to be left entirely to parents." Natural selection apparently thought so, too.

For helping mothers, especially in parts of the world where resources are scarce, the nearby presence of a grandmother increases the child's chance for survival. This is true in tribal communities in Africa, India, and South America as well as in European and North American farming communities, with a possible caveat that the grandmothers not be overwhelmingly needy themselves. Among the Khasi tribal people in northeast India, for example, anthropologists found that the chances of a child's dying were 74% greater if he or she did not have a grandmother living with the family. Hrdy explains that "Experienced in childcare, sensitive to infant cues, adept at local subsistence tasks, undistracted by babies of their own or even the possibility of having them, and (like old men as well) repositories of useful knowledge, postmenopausal females are also unusually altruistic."

We have evolved to introduce the father's resources as well. Many evolutionary biologists now think that the father's central involvement in the baby's care increases not only his or her chance of survival but also his or her overall success in life. Over the course of evolution, not only would a father's empathic skills help parents determine why a baby was crying, and thus directly help the baby survive, but indirectly such skills also helped the baby form alliances and secure mates.

With fathers' increasing role in childrearing, they became more interested in keeping tabs on who exactly their own kids were. Their heightened interest provided an incentive to form committed relationships with women. In fact, De Waal points out that the size of human testicles—tiny in comparison to many apes'—can be taken as a sign that humans are made to commit. Because a man is unlikely to share his mate with others, he does not need to give her an overdose of sperm to maximize his chances of winning the race against another man's sperm. A little bit of sperm will do. By comparison, chimps—who freely, openly, and regularly change mates—have testicles ten times bigger than those of humans, after correcting for relative body size. Bonobos, which are even more promiscuous than chimps, have the testicles to prove it. As De Waal states, "Our anatomy tells a story of romance and bonding between the sexes going back a long time, perhaps to the very beginnings of our lineage."

De Waal and other biologists offer us a tidy evolutionary narrative for the evolution of altruism. Commitment gave rise to the nuclear family and the nuclear family, in turn, had a major calming effect on men. Because most adult men were then nearly guaranteed sex, they no longer had to compete for it with other men (the major source of conflict in most ape communities). Thus, according to De Waal's evolutionary account, without this source of strife, men were able to use their big brains to start cooperating with one another in a reciprocal manner, working together to get that stag, and ultimately build societies.

Even Machines Can Evolve Cooperative Strategies

We think of evolution as applying primarily to biological organisms, but "evolution" as an idea actually applies to an array of entities and processes. (If you search Google under "evolution of," the algorithm quickly suggests "evolution of dance" and "evolution of the hipster"— neither exactly applies here, but both results make my point). Because Chapter 2 examines straightforward *physical mechanisms* for producing altruistic behaviors, we can derive comfort from tangible evidence that no "religious capacity" or "supernatural faculty" is necessary for good behavior. Because machines could never have a religious capacity, their ability to evolve cooperative strategies is particularly interesting, suggesting that the altruism involved in cooperation comes from the needs of the entity itself, and does not somehow need an external stimulant, source, or reference. Long ago, cooperation was shown in computer simulations to be beneficial in the long run to the computers themselves. The classic example of this phenomenon is a controversial game called Tit for Tat, a simple and "cooperative" computer program that was created in the late 1970s by Anatol Rapoport.

Rapoport set up each Tit for Tat computer game to start by cooperating with its partner and then to do whatever its "partner" did last. In this simple program, cooperation begets cooperation. If the partner defects (i.e., departs from a cooperative strategy) the program also defects. If the partner then cooperates, the program forgives and cooperates. Despite its simple two lines of code, Tit for Tat swept aside all other programs in Robert Axelrod's computer tournaments playing iterative Prisoner's Dilemma, a classic game of trust meant to model actual human interaction. By "swept aside" I mean that Tit for Tat achieved an evolutionarily stable status that lasted, whereas other computerized approaches did not. Please note that the idea behind the prisoner's dilemma is that you find yourself isolated from a partner—perhaps a partner in crime, the way the classic story is usually told—and are faced with two options: cooperate or defect. If you choose "cooperate" and your partner chooses "cooperate," you both get, say, $300. If you cooperate and your partner defects you get nothing and he gets $500. Or vice versa. If you both defect, you both get $100. Obviously, it is to your advantage to defect—but your partner likely understands the same logic. And if you both defect, the payoff is less than if you both cooperate. Key point: there is no way of knowing what the other will do, so the mutually cooperative strategy is the safest strategy, long term. Tit for Tat's success has been used to show that cooperation, once it emerges, is a viable and powerful strategy for survival—one that may have swept other strategies aside. Remember, there is no human mind or reference to religious authority involved here. A computer program—a machine—can achieve mutual cooperation. Mechanisms in the brain can as well.

In his 1984 book, *The Evolution of Cooperation*, Axelrod is careful to stress that the success of the Tit for Tat decision rule likely rested on the expected repeated interaction of individuals. This, in conjunction with the understanding that we lived in relatively small societies until only a few thousand years ago, has been used as an argument to keep communities and even companies small so as to increase the likelihood of repeated interactions with the same individuals and, thereby, foster innate tendencies for cooperation.

Though this seems like a sensible view, a recent study showed that our tendency to act in a reciprocal manner is even more robust than Axelrod implied. In 2011, a team of scientists conducted a series of computer simulations designed to test if evolution would really select against goodwill in situations where future interaction (and thus payoff) was improbable. Surprising biologists and economists, their work showed that acting to help others, even when there are no foreseeable repeated interactions, "emerges naturally." They explain that this is due to the inherent unpredictability of social life—maybe you will run into that taxi driver again—as well as the relative low cost of acting with kindness. Their finding supports that altruism is not the product of social pressure, but is instead a fundamental part of human nature.

And Mind Your Reputation

Still another phenomenon that likely shaped our tendency to be generous—instinctively and naturally—may at first seem counterintuitive, considering that we all frequently (and guiltily) indulge in this phenomenon: "gossip." So-called gossip may be partly responsible for shaping humans into the do-gooders they are today.

Randolph Nesse, who also practices as a psychiatrist, has compellingly theorized that our ability to make commitments to one another has underpinned most of human development. Commitments, in turn, are largely underscored by reputation. And "reputation" is really just a nice word for all the gossip concerning one individual and whether or not, and how much, gossip actually exists. Whom should a guy ask along on a stag hunt? Whom would you trust to do well by you in a foxhole or in some other difficult situation?

So now let's add language skills to a man's or woman's "toolkit" of trust assessment. Suddenly, our hunter has more to draw upon than just his own experiences. With chatter, he can listen and learn about the experiences others have had with "prospective hunter friend." As a result, he can estimate this potential buddy's reputation as a hard worker and a generous divider of game. Obviously, those known to exhibit kindness and cooperation always would have been favored by the community and thus by Nature. Those who had poor reputations, who were regarded as shirkers or hoarders, won few partnerships and were pushed to the outskirts of the group. Adding language skills makes this expulsion process faster, and less forgiving.

In 2000, Nowak and Sigmond created a computer simulation of cooperation that modeled the importance of reputation even in single interactions. They observed that "The evolution of human language as a means of such information transfer [i.e., gossip about past actions] has certainly helped in the emergence of cooperation." Nesse further explains that "So long as each player's reputation is revealed sufficiently, cooperation can grow."

Evolution of Grammar in Relation to Our "Hard-wired" Altruism

Starting with a seminal book in 1957, MIT linguist Noam Chomsky argued that we are innately wired to form grammatical sentences. Does the wiring for altruistic behavior that I will illustrate in Chapter 2 pre-date the wiring for grammar? Most likely, parts of the brain known to be involved in speech production and comprehension are located in the relatively recently evolved frontal lobes, while the wiring for beneficent behavior most definitely involves ancient structures such as the amygdala, a complex set of nerve cell groups deep beneath the brain's cortex. Basically, by analogy, even as Chomsky argued that we are "hard wired" for producing grammatical sentences, I argue that we are "hard wired" for producing altruistic behaviors. We are both talking about how specific neuronal connections underlie basic human behaviors. Though beneficent behavior likely evolved first, its wiring was likely strengthened with language development because of the "reputation factor" that we just discussed. If higher primates can express *what's the news* concerning various potential friends and scoundrels, then use of mechanisms for social behavior will be improved—made more socially efficient—for the benefit of the individual and group.

Pointedly, a recent study by psychologist Eric Anderson and colleagues demonstrated that we pay more attention to the face of a person whom we've heard gossip about, even if the face is presented in a way that precludes our ability to be consciously aware of it. That is, expressing interest in a face occurs even before our conscious recognition of that face. The capacity for gossip likely strengthened our primate tendency to want to make sure that we are in each other's good graces—because not only is everyone paying attention, but one slip-up and everyone will know. And group displeasure could literally be a death sentence.

De Waal states that "Fear of ostracism lurks in the corners of every human mind." We share this fear with our closest cousins, as nonhuman primates in general and humans cannot survive on their own for long. This is why primates devote so much time—up to 10% of each day—to maintaining and strengthening social ties by grooming others. The human equivalent to grooming, he says, is small talk.

Of course, while we all exchange news and share our feelings, many biologists have pointed out that the best way to appear honest and kind is actually to *be* honest and kind. As Nesse points out, because we evolved in small kin groups, helping others usually helped our own genes, and so it was more cost effective to just be kind, rather than to calculate advantages. Even today, friends are likely to have similar genotypes, according to Fowler and his group. While in evolutionary terms we have only recently begun living in large societies, the instinctive drive toward behaving with goodwill has stayed with us.

Moreover, as predicted by the computer programs such as Axelrod's, reciprocally altruistic behavior is the secret to our success. Once reciprocity got a foothold with cooperative breeding, the various benefits of acting with goodwill caused runaway selection for those who just couldn't help acting in a reciprocally altruistic fashion. These benefits are not only what makes us human, but also have given rise to all the unique attributes that make humanity so interesting, powerful, and effective. They are also critical to our continued survival. James Duffy, Professor of Psychiatry at the University of Texas, and Fellow of the McGovern Center for Health, Healing, and the Human Spirit, has observed that: "It is reasonable to suggest the evolution of human beings has occurred as a consequence of our neural capacity to create and support trusting and affiliative relationships across broader and broader domains of social connectivity. Whilst the social groups of the earliest humans included their immediate clan, post-modern humans must continually create these affiliative relationships with individuals with whom they may never have significant indirect physical contact." I would only add that over vast stretches of their history, humans have *practiced* the formation of such broad-gauge, beneficial relationships.

Is There Evolutionary Discontinuity to Human Brains that Are Wired for Good Behavior?

In his recent book, *The Tell-Tale Brain*, V. S. Ramachandran tries to make a strong case for the disconnection between the brains of nonhuman primates and the human brain. While he is not comfortable with simple dichotomous questions like "Are humans 'just' animals or are we exalted?," in his chapter "No Mere Ape" he emphasizes the role of culture as "a significant new source of evolutionary pressure" in producing unique features of human behavior. Of course, for my argument, the ability to produce language is not part of the discussion because we are focusing on the capacity for social recognition and affiliation. Emphasizing the tremendous complexity of the connections among neurons in our cerebral cortex, Ramachandran talks about "a new pathway, highly developed in humans" that serves the analysis of visual scenes. As to how new connections contribute to human uniqueness, he argues that the "liberation from the constraints of a strictly gene-based Darwinian evolution" constitutes a "giant step in human evolution."

Quite beyond questions of linguistic ability, I can imagine arguments in favor of Ramachandran's point of view. Mathematics, of course, is not associated with the behaviors of baboons and chimpanzees. Though some might consider mathematics somewhat similar to language, I would claim that within human populations, individual differences in math and language do not vary relative to each other—those of us who are best at one are not necessarily best at the other.

The literature on animal behavior is rife with examples of golden-rule–like behavior among nonhuman primates, the most famous being reports by De Waal about the dispositions of bonobos, sophisticated primates with abilities similar to those of chimpanzees, toward civilized social organization. More recently, Joan Silk described prosocial behavior among female baboons, saying that mutual grooming and close cooperative contact with other members of the group actually conferred a reproductive advantage. Hans Kummer reviewed some of the older literature on nonhuman primates, giving examples of altruistic behavior ranging from food sharing, sexual fidelity, and respecting another's social relationship, to helping a relative under attack. Altruistic habits such as these among non-human primates make the universality, of golden rule–producing neuronal circuits among human societies, easier to accept.

The strongest claim for animal/human discontinuity that I have been able to find was published recently by a multi-university team headed by anthropologist Kim Hill, who cooperated in this effort with scientists from the United States and Ethiopia. Hill explained that "because we humans have lived as foragers for 95% of our species history," this large team studied present-day foraging societies, 32 of them, comprising a total sample of 5067 individuals. A foraging society was defined as a group that gets its food by hunting and gathering. They found "that hunter-gatherers display a unique social structure" where either males or females can disperse among subgroups, adult siblings often co-reside, and "most individuals in residential groups are genetically unrelated." The authors argue that "these patterns (of residence) produce large interaction networks of unrelated adults," and as a result foster extensive cooperation that contributes to the success of the human species. Such cooperation includes widespread sharing of food, taking care of other families' babies, and the construction and maintenance of living spaces. The complex and flexible structures of alliances permitted by Hill's findings can be contrasted to the simple single-group structures of other primate societies. We do not know how this unique human social structure evolved, but it evidently led to economic and other biological or psychological benefits that permitted our species' relative success.

Geneticist Francisco Ayala goes further. He thinks that humans have a moral sense not present in other species, because humans have all "three necessary conditions for ethical behavior: anticipation of the consequences of one's actions, the ability to make value judgments, and the ability to choose between alternative courses of action." Chapter 2 argues that lower animals also have all three of these capacities, as long as you'll allow me to say that "making a value judgment" can be afforded by an animal's being able to distinguish between consequences that are emotionally good and emotionally bad. Sentimentally, it is easy to relax and accept Ayala's opinion that humans are quite special, but I am frustrated by anthropologists and others like Professor Ramachandran, who claim "distinctive origins" for human social behaviors, especially altruistic behaviors, without providing proof.

Ayala and others have underestimated the social capacities of nonhuman primates' capacities, which allow us to claim that there is a continuous enrichment of social behaviors as we move from nonhuman primate to human, with the big leaps due to language. Consider Frans De Waal's study, "Giving is self-rewarding for monkeys." In various trials, he observed that monkeys chose responses that would get food for neighboring, familiar, visible monkeys more frequently than they would evince "selfish" responses that provided food only for themselves. The more the experiment went on, the more frequently they chose the generous option, suggesting that being generous and prosocial was reinforcing to them. In trials in which the subject monkeys chose the generous option, they liked to turn and orient themselves toward the recipient monkey, suggesting that they enjoyed seeing the result of their generous act. The subject monkeys understood the nature of their act, and enjoyed seeing the other monkeys receiving food as a result of their act.

Along these same lines, Victoria Horner, working with De Waal, performed an experiment in which chimpanzees were given tokens that could be exchanged for food. One color of token would get the test chimp some food, but the other color meant that a chimp in another cage would get food as well. The results showed that the test chimps used the color that would get another chimp food (in addition to itself) significantly more often than the "selfish, exclusive" color of token. Horner said that this type of altruistic behavior matched the type of generous behavior she had seen among chimps in the wild.

Biologists frequently underestimate the abilities of higher animals. From my perspective, it is clear that those animals can do everything that scientists have already seen that they can do, plus those animals can do more; they have sensory and motor capacities, an ability to learn complex skills, and still others to perform complex tasks. Based on the trajectory of our knowledge, we are likely to learn that they can also do many more such things. But in animals as in humans, certain abilities shine only under particular circumstances. The most fortunate environments allow the animal to really show you everything it can do, whereas bad circumstances lead to below-par behavior. Picture the remarkable abilities of a nonhuman primate imagined in the movie *Rise of the Planet of the Apes*, where James Franco's character brings an ape from the lab to lead an ape revolution. Refusing to underestimate the social capacities of nonhuman primates, I suspect that with regard to basic altruistic capacities, the similarities between humans and other primates are more impressive than any differences. Indeed, as Morris B. Hoffman has argued: "Although no contemporary non-human primates seem to have moral systems quite like ours, they have all the behavioral ingredients necessary—attachment, bonding, cooperation, defection, defection-detection, and empathy—for [what has been] called 'pre-moral sentiments.' Reciprocal altruism is itself a kind of pre-moral sentiment, requiring the ability to give an accept benefits with an anticipation of a promised return."

Scientists will have still more warnings for those who celebrate the uniqueness of human social behaviors. Those who claim uniqueness for human behaviors must always point to a discontinuity, that is, a "jump" from nonhuman to human. Such a jump simply means the lack of an intermediate case. It is always dangerous for a scientist to argue from an *absence* of evidence. Next week or next year, that dispositive intermediate case may be discovered, and the "discontinuity to the human brain" discarded.

Consider the evidence from paleoanthropology and genetics. Using the logic just cited, it is impossible to prove the "unique human brain" argument by looking back over eons, while it is easy to favor "continuity" while just waiting for the intermediate cases show up. In addition, it would seem that the greater the number of early hominid species that populated the earth—especially Africa, where our modern human species is supposed to have arisen—the greater the probability that one of them was on the line to the evolutionarily intermediate brain state. In fact, geneticists are now discovering more archaic hominid species than were previously supposed to have existed in Africa, and they believe that there may have been more interbreeding than was previously suspected. Further, British paleoanthropologist Chris Stringer also thinks that Africa today has "the greatest internal genetic variation of any inhabited continent," and he has been quoted as saying that more early hominid species were simultaneously roaming around the land mass than had previously been thought. Such paleoanthropologic findings, taken together with those of genetics, reveal that the scene was more complicated and heterogeneous than we thought; it offers an array of opportunities for the continuous development of brain and behavior, rather than supporting the sudden emergence of a "unique human brain." The paleoanthropologist will always argue for evolutionary continuity, and so will I.

As a supporter of continuity, I argue that the human brain is different than that of nonhuman primates only as a matter of degree, at least with respect to social behaviors. Nevertheless, as evolutionary psychologist Micheal Tomasello puts it, "To an unprecedented degree, homo sapiens are adapted for acting and thinking cooperatively in cultural groups, and indeed all of humans' most impressive cognitive achievements—from complex technologies to linguistic and mathematical symbols to intricate social institutions—are the products not of individuals acting alone, but of individuals interacting."

In the brain, such selection pressures caused the development of powerful neural mechanisms for empathy and goodwill that were uncovered over the last couple of decades. For now, suffice it to say, we have shown that genes known to promote mating and parenting behavior are also necessary for basic social skills such as learning from those outside one's kin—a skill that makes cooperation and, indeed, society, possible. In sum, before hominids were quite human—but already possessed some ability to feel the pain of others and take another's perspective similarly to the abilities of other modern Great Apes—they stumbled into a niche that we can each individually benefit from inhabiting if we all work (and create blood banks and teach babies) together. The original pressure for this coordination among humans came, not from without—that is, not necessarily from competitive war-like apes who cooperated to attack other apes—but rather from within, from our own children and loved ones. From there, instinctual behavior and brain activity that evolved to aid cooperative breeding spilled into other areas of our lives, giving rise to altruistic behavior and causing us to act with goodwill even toward strangers.

The point is that behaviors that seem to indicate "empathy" can be found in nature—not just in modern humans—and we have evolved to make the most of our own empathic qualities. Consider this sweeping statement by James Duffy:

> It is fair to state that empathy has been the social bootstrap that has supported the emergence of increasingly complex societies. Empathy is essential for maternal nurturance and the establishment of maternal bonds....
>
> Several recent paleontological findings indicate that Neanderthals and middle Pleistocene hominins provided nurturant and compassionate care to disabled members of their clan. Furthermore, primates and even rodents and birds have been reported to exhibit altruistic behaviors to con-specifics. [Researchers] in the "social brain hypothesis" suggested that increasingly complex social environments are the primary selective pressure for the explosive growth of the human brain over the past few millennia.

We should think of our capacity for empathy as embedded in an evolutionary process that, though not unique to humans, has allowed humans to create societies that, as a consequence, have enabled our species to thrive.

Having discussed how altruistic mechanisms evolved, this book will now address how such mechanisms can work in the human brain. Indeed, it is possible to specify steps in nerve cell operations that theoretically produce reciprocal altruistic behaviors in humans.

FURTHER READING

Robert Axelrod. 1984. *The Evolution of Cooperation*. New York: Basic Books.

Dorothy Cheney. 2011. "Extent and Limits of Cooperation in Animals." *PNAS* 108, Suppl. 2, 10902–10909.

Richard Dawkins. 2006. *The Selfish Gene*. Oxford: Oxford University Press (first published 1976).

Frans De Waal. 2010. *The Age of Empathy*. London: Souvenir Press.

Oren Harman. 2010. *The Price of Altruism*. New York: W. W. Norton.

V. Horner, J. Carter, J., M. Suchak, and F. de Waal. 2011. "Spontaneous Prosocial Choice by Chimpanzees." *PNAS* 108, Suppl. 2, 13847–13851.

Sarah Hrdy. 2009. *Mothers and Others*. Cambridge, MA: The Belknap Press.

Martin Nowak with R. Highfield. 2011. *SuperCooperators: The Mathematics of Evolution, Altruism, and Human Behavior*. New York: Free Press.

V. S. Ramachandran. 2011. *The Tell-Tale Brain: A Neuroscientist's Quest for What Makes Us Human*. New York: W. W. Norton.

Robert Seyfarth and Dorothy Cheney. 2012. "The Evolutionary Origins of Friendship," *Annual Review of Psychology* 63. Palo Alto: Annual Reviews, 179–199.

J. Silk and B. House. 2011. "Evolutionary Foundations of Human Prosocial Sentiments," *PNAS* 108, Suppl. 2, 10910–10917.

J. Strassmann, D. Queller, J. Avise, and F. Ayala. 2011. "In the Light of Evolution, Volume V: Cooperation and Conflict" *PNAS* 108, Suppl. 2, 10787–10791.

C. Stringer. 2012. *Lone Survivors*. New York: Henry Holt.

Michael Tomasello. 2009. *Why We Cooperate*. Cambridge, MA: MIT Press.

Edward O. Wilson. 2012. *The Social Conquest of Earth*. New York: W. W. Norton.

[2]

ALTRUISTIC BRAIN THEORY INTRODUCED

So far, we have examined biological approaches to how reciprocal altruism evolved over several millennia. The narrative is a timeline of hard scientific evidence that describes how humans' basic instincts— parenthood, sex—led even the earliest people to become unalterably communal. It was human instinct wired into our brains that enabled us to form crucial bonds, to care for each other because it seemed natural and because communities offered a form of well-being superior to that felt by remaining on one's own. In terms of explaining how *Homo sapiens* got to be recognizably human, therefore, no single approach is more powerful than evolution. Humans feature complexes of personality traits that have stood the test of time and allowed them to develop a basic, shared, indeed universal personality substrate. The point of dwelling on "evolutionary biology" for an entire chapter was thus to demonstrate that altruism is not something that humans recently learned as life became more "civilized." To extend the theme further, it is also not something that we discovered along with the development of religious morality. Altruism is as much a part of us as the desire for a mate or concern to protect our children. We do not have to think about it when the occasion presents, just as we don't have to think about whether sex is interesting. It just is.

But just as evolutionary biology is essentially a trajectory of how-we-got-here-from-there, so is of the idea of Altruistic Brain Theory (ABT), albeit on a much compressed timescale. How, over the course of some few hundredths of a second, do our brains make us swing into action to help another person? This book explains altruistic behavior for the first time by reviewing hundreds of scientific papers that coalesce into support for a five-step theory of how altruistic action occurs. It does not "just happen;" rather, we are unconscious of discrete *steps* that our brains take to bring us to that point. Part of our evolutionary adaptation is that our brains do not stop to reflect when we are about to be altruistic; if they did, we might not act, as sometimes altruism involves personal risk. Think, for example, of Wesley Autrey, or the school personnel in Newtown, Connecticut who jumped on top of five- and six-year-olds in their charge to shield them from a rampaging gunman. Nonetheless, there is a series of definable, neuronal/hormonal activities that our brains undertake before we can actually behave altruistically. Until now, neuroscientists have described elements of a mosaic that, had they been assembled in just the right order, might have constituted a similar theory. Yet though the constituent knowledge was available in the literature, no one ever made the leap. ABT thus represents the first time that our knowledge has been synthesized into a comprehensive neuroscientific approach to altruism.

An historian or philosopher of science might ask why, when knowledge of the brain has been accruing for decades, no one ever saw how the pieces could fit together into a *brain mechanism* for altruism. Why didn't anyone even try? As stated in the Introduction, there were plenty of institutional reasons why scientists might have shied away from this topic. Among those were neuroscientists' needs to attack easier and clearly solvable problems. Plus, scientists are eager to show quantifiable results. It may also have been because scientists always cited evolution when they sought to explain altruism. Hence the question got pigeonholed in evolutionary biology.

But evolution, which is crucial for demonstrating that the biological sources of human altruism have run deep through time, does not explain how altruism actually works, right now, on a neuronal/hormonal level. In *The Neurophysiology of Mind*, the Nobel Prize winner Sir John Eccles speculated that God somehow designed the brain to produce altruistic behavior. But that is simply not a scientific theory. Accordingly, while I wish that I could say that I am intervening in a vigorous scientific debate about how brain mechanisms produce empathy and altruism, in fact there is very little debate because the problem has not been the focus of research. Lately, the psychologist Richard Davidson, who is discussed later in this book, has shown that if we practice morality the brain will actually develop pathways that reinforce that behavior. This is an important insight and draws attention to the connection between morality and brain mechanisms. But even Davidson does not broach the idea that the mechanisms for moral behavior exist in our brains from the day that we are born. What I want to do now, therefore, is to demonstrate how all the latest science leads us to specific, definable neuronal/hormonal mechanisms that necessarily entail altruism, such that mechanisms for altruism are literally built into the brain.

ABT explains exactly how altruistic behavior happens when it happens. The theory comprises a surprising convergence of decades of neurophysiological evidence gathered in laboratories all over the world. My expertise in this area comes from producing and studying data from several areas of neuroscience—neuroanatomy, neurophysiology, behavioral neuroscience, and molecular neuroendocrinology—and bringing them together in ABT, which explains the best, most prosocial features of the vast majority of human social behaviors. But how does it work?

This chapter, therefore, asks (and answers) this question: *What brain mechanisms operate to impel us toward mutual concern, and indeed toward a virtually instinctive disposition toward acting on those concerns?*

In the simplest terms, how do we accomplish the altruistic acts that nature programmed us to perform? It is crucial that we understand this "how" if only as an exercise in self-exploration. Humans are curious about themselves, and the brain is our most complex organ, one that affects every other organ in our bodies. To understand the brain—to appreciate it—is therefore not just for neuroscientists. At the other extreme, neither is it just for philosophers who seek to extend our understanding of the brain into theories of how we experience the world. If the average person would have a basic understanding of metabolism, sleep, and other physiological functions (which, by the way, the brain controls), why shouldn't he seek to understand at least one phase of how the brain orders the moral equivalent of these basic functions, what we might call their temperament? Obviously, he should.

As a corollary, if we are ever to systematically address our own self-improvement, then knowing where in the brain to start would obviously be necessary. Social engineers come in every stripe imaginable, but they are all mostly hortatory, appealing to everyone's desire to live in a better world without yet getting down to the one organ that actually controls behavior. Of course, culture is indeed a *backdrop* to any aspirational activity, but starting with the brain provides the sort of instant credibility that, say, an abstract appeal to "fighting poverty" does not. We can all agree on the brain, and an understanding of its functions can help us agree on addressing our shared, human concerns in a way that is as culture-neutral as it is possible to be.

Moreover, by realizing how the brain naturally favors altruistic behavior, we can bolster our confidence in humanity's own best instincts, as well as society's confidence in the various social tools that rely on trust. (I discuss these in Chapter 7.) When you look around right now, be it at our squabbling Congress or the various rogue nations developing atomic weapons, it is easy to be pessimistic about ever improving the human condition. But there is still a great deal in all of us that can inspire hope. ABT seeks to establish a degree of scientific reliability in our expectations about human behavior. If we can count on ourselves to display an instinctive altruism—if altruism is our default position—then we can potentially believe that cultural differences are not insurmountable, and that the brain holds out the promise of our working together. As I observed in Chapter 1, such "working together" is how we were *wired* to behave as we evolved. Indeed, ABT is powerfully predictive of how our brains will compel us, over the long haul and in the great majority of instances, to behave well toward one another, both individually and in groups. Altruism will carry the day. As a species, it is our destiny. We cannot allow ourselves to become stymied by the outcrop of bad, even egregious behavior. In the aggregate, we are *going* to display socially useful traits. The point is to develop mechanisms, personal and social, to harness this built-in proclivity. As this book demonstrates, ABT can provide the basis for new initiatives that clear away the impediments to prosocial behavior and allow people to perform *on a regular basis* in accordance with their potential.

This is not a blithely futuristic claim. This book contends that if bad behavior represents a very small proportion of people's actions, then ABT explains the rest—that is, all the tremendous amounts of good behavior. It does so, furthermore, without making extraordinary assumptions about the brain's reasoning abilities. Step by inexorable step, the theory shows how the brain produces altruistic behavior in quite a surprising way: not by relying on greater information processing than usual, but by actually cutting back on the precision of the information flow. Actually, ABT theory says that we do "more" with less overall data.

This chapter will therefore do three things. First and most importantly, it will lay out the details of ABT. Second, it will provide a glimpse of the large amounts of neuroscientific evidence that proves each step and that will be explained in detail Chapter 3. Third, to follow the details of ABT in terms of a real-life event, we will consider a striking example: Stephen Siller. Siller, an experienced New York City fireman, was going to play golf with his brothers on his day off, September 11, 2001. He was in Brooklyn. When he learned about a plane hitting one of the Twin Towers, he drove to the Brooklyn Battery Tunnel, ran through it carrying more than 50 pounds of firefighting gear, and made his way as quickly as possible into Manhattan. Once there, another fireman brought him to the towers, where he died during a rescue attempt. So how do we explain Siller's altruism, as well as that of 343 other firefighters and first responders who lost their lives on 9/11 trying to help others? What are the brain mechanisms of such incredible altruism, and of millions of everyday acts of kindness?

ABT tells us that within a few hundredths of a second after we realize a need for action our brains will make the decision for altruistic behavior. It's hard to imagine that it all happens so fast, but the entire task of neuroscience is to analyze and describe what is essentially imperceptible in real time. In this sense, neuroscience is unlike, say, cardiology or most medical disciplines, which can literally watch the body in real time as it functions. In neuroscience, we have to understand the brain's deep structures and functions, and describe what is virtually impossible to capture in a stop-time photograph. *The brain is that fast.* It is in this mode, describing what we can illustrate in a diagram but cannot see as it unfolds, that I present the steps of ABT, together with just a "snapshot" of the scientific proof cited in the next chapter. Moreover, because the steps identified in ABT issue in an action—rather than, say, an ongoing physical condition—the theory has an abstract quality that does not lend itself to the examining table. But if you think about it, it's in this very sense that it shares in the basic aspect of how we live most of our lives. That is, we *don't* examine the vast majority our actions in advance. So it is in this everyday sense that I present the theory, which comes in five definable steps.

STEP 1: REPRESENTATION OF WHAT THE PERSON (IN THIS CASE, SILLER) IS ABOUT TO DO

This step of ABT does not merely rely on just one study or one lab's work to support it. Rather, it is proven by an entire field of neurophysiology called corollary discharge, summarized in Chapter 3 and introduced here.

Electrophysiological research going back to 1947 proves that virtually all neuronal signals sent from the brain or spinal cord to the muscles to produce a body movement have a copy. These copies are sent over to the relevant sensory systems so that the brain knows what is about to happen. In our September 11, 2011 example, however, Siller's impending act (running to the towers) will unconsciously be represented in his brain before he can carry it out. Here's how that happens. The same nerve cells at the top of the neural system that will command the muscles to contract (and hence undertake the act) also send a second, identical message back to the sensory systems of the brain that essentially says "these muscles are about to contract in this exact manner." While it's perhaps easiest to understand the capacity to send this second, identical electrical signal (called "corollary discharge") from parts of the cerebral cortex controlling movement (the "motor cortex"), many other parts of the brain directing motor activity are capable of doing the same thing: this includes a large motor control zone in the forebrain beneath the cortex, the cerebellum, and the hindbrain. All of these motor control zones are known to cooperate in the production (and registering) of coordinated movement.

In the meantime, however, "corollary discharge" serves perfectly as the first step of ABT, and has become an ordinary part of our understanding of neurophysiology. Corollary discharges from the motor controls to sensory systems are required for our perception that the world is "holding still"—is physically in the same place despite our bodily movement—because such discharges allow our brains to predict changes in the world that are consequent to each of our behaviors. That is, as a result of this second motor signal, the brain knows what the body is about to do.

It is important to note that this first step is not particular to ABT, but is rather an ordinary part of everyday neurophysiology. Unless one's act toward another person is represented to one's central nervous system, the potential effect of that act on the other person cannot be evaluated in Step 4. In ABT, the representation of our incipient behavior leads naturally to Step 2, perceiving the social object of that behavior.

STEP 2: PERCEPTION OF THE INDIVIDUAL TOWARD WHOM THE BENEFACTOR (IN THIS CASE SILLER) WILL ACT

A major development in neurophysiological research has been the explanation of exactly how we perceive the visual world. Of course, when we look at the object of our intended social action we cannot avoid perceiving him or her. Here and in Chapter 3, I will summarize the evidence from the field of visual physiology that leads inevitably to ABT Step 2.

Hundreds of scientific papers describe how our brains perceive the visual world around us. Patterns of light pass through our eyes to cause corresponding patterns of nerve cell excitation on the retinas in the backs of our eyes. Those electrical signals race up the optic nerve and then either turn toward our midbrain, where a simplified version of the visual pattern triggers a rapid, reflex action, or go to the thalamus, where the really detailed visual processing begins. "Thalamus" is the Greek word for "antechamber" and is called that because the thalamus is the obligatory processing station for visual signals to enter the cortex. When Siller is about to act toward a wounded person in the tower, he brings to mind a vision of a (generic) person in the tower. Neurons in the visual part of Siller's brain fire in patterns that represent the image of such a person, who represents large numbers of actual people in the tower. (While a benefactor frequently sees the object of his intended action right in front of him, in other cases the visual cortex simply registers a vision of a distant or even hypothetical person, in this case, a generic person in the tower.) In our example, Siller's brain processes the visual information that creates an image of a generic tower victim. In other cases, when the actual beneficiary is right in front of the benefactor, the patterns of light, dark, and color that pass through the eyes of the actor (the person who is about to behave, i.e., the benefactor) cause electrical signals to be sent from the cells of the retina; the signals travel through the optic nerve. As I mentioned, the signals follow two major pathways. The simpler, more primitive pathway heads for the midbrain, where visual signals can be put together with signals from other senses to get a rapid picture of what is in front of the actor and enable rapid, almost automatic action. The longer, more detailed visual pathway special to the human brain travels to the very top of the brainstem, thus to signal to the very back of the cerebral cortex, the visual cortex. There, individual features of the image of the other person—lines, angles, shadows—converge in groups of cells to form a unified image. Neuron by neuron, these lines and angles are encoded, as shown by the Nobel Prize–winning work of Torsten Wiesel (former president of Rockefeller University) as he worked at Harvard with David Hubel.

Step 2 is crucial to ABT because we cannot act toward another human being unless we can literally picture that person—or visualize a generic person—in all of his or her humanity. This is part of the communal impulse programmed into us by evolution, and necessary for our survival. Apart from the bare physiological mechanisms that make up Step 2, it is *understandable* and even necessary in evolutionary terms.

STEP 3: MERGE IMAGES OF THE VICTIM WHOM SILLER WILL HELP WITH SILLER'S OWN SELF-IMAGE

Step 3 is the most novel for neuroscience, unique to ABT, and is crucial for ABT to work properly. It represents a new insight, and a different way of thinking about how the brain produces altruistic behavior. While each nerve cell mechanism mentioned here and illustrated in Chapter 3 is grounded in hundreds of scientific papers, ABT brings them together in a single theory.

In everyone's brain a set of firing nerve cells constitutes a unified image of the person toward whom one will act, as well as a neural image of oneself. (We always have an image of ourselves in our brain). The question for Step 3 of ABT is: how exactly could the image of another person be linked, constantly overlapped with our own image? The answer is: an increase in the excitability of cortical neurons, such that when the nerve cells representing the other are firing signals, the nerve cells representing self are also firing.

How might this cross-excitation of images happen in the cerebral cortex? There are three cellular mechanisms that can do this. One is that inhibition in the cortex is reduced (for details, see Chapter 3). A second mechanism is that tiny tunnels between nerve cells are created, thus allowing electrical excitation to spread quickly. A third mechanism implicates excitation by the powerful neurotransmitter acetylcholine. In addition to these three mechanisms for merging sensory images of other with self, the so-called mirror neurons unite the actions of another person with our own. My mirror neurons that signal I will raise my right hand fire signals when you raise your right hand; in this way, such mirror neurons can be thought of as supporting my empathy for you. So a multiplicity of nerve cell mechanisms underlies the merging of your image with mine, as we shall see in Step 4.

But as frequently happens in the brain, we are not dealing with processes that are distinct or mutually exclusive. Rather, all of these mechanisms for merging images can work in parallel, and can assume different relative importance in different individuals. ABT takes advantage of the brain's redundancies, its capacity to do things in different ways, sometimes in many ways at once. Of course, this type of multifaceted capability makes sense from an evolutionary standpoint, because if one capacity goes down another will still be available. But for my purposes, it also means that ABT does not at this stage have to rely on one or another process, as humans have built-in overcapacities to perform even the simplest mental tasks.

In our 9/11 example, Siller visualizes a wounded person in the Twin Towers. Whereas it is extremely difficult for the brain to keep these visual images separate and distinct, it is *extremely easy* for them to get mixed up with each other; that mix-up or "blurring" of images is precisely what is needed for an efficient theory of altruistic behavior. To put it another way, in the brain of the person who will initiate the act toward another person, the difference between the target person's image and his own will unconsciously be brought to zero. Where there is a discrete image of the target in the cerebral cortex and elsewhere, and another discrete image of the target person, the brain now produces a merged image where images of the two persons coalesce. Step 3 is important because unless the two images are merged in the cerebral cortex, the image of the "other" cannot be treated like the "self." Chapter 3 will show four separate brain mechanisms by which this can happen.

STEP 4: THE ALTRUISTIC BRAIN

A long tradition of research on the functions of the prefrontal cortex shows how the outputs from Steps 1 and 3 arrive at neurons whose activities produce the Altruistic Brain. That is, the representation of the act (from Step 1) and the united, combined image (from Step 3) must arrive at an "ethical switch" in the brain just before we carry out an act toward another person. As a result, instead of literally seeing the consequences of the act for another person, we automatically envision the consequences as pertaining to our own self! For example, Siller acted in a way that he would have wanted someone to act toward him if he were in the Twin Towers. While this ethical evaluation may occur at a conscious level, it also can be instantaneous and unconscious.

Where in the brain does this juncture of the act's representation with the combined image of self and other take place? Based on current neuroscience, the best conclusion is that it takes place primarily in a part of the brain that is bigger and stronger in the human brain than in other brains: the prefrontal cortex (see Figure 2.1). The work of Joshua Greene, covered in Chapter 5, highlights the activation of neurons in the prefrontal cortex during the making of moral decisions. There, a value—"good" or "bad," "do" or "don't do"—is attached to the combination of the act and the combined self/other

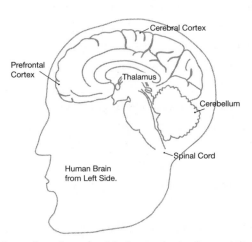

Figure 2.1 The prefrontal cortex of the human brain plays an important role in Altruistic Brain function.

target. These prefrontal cortical neurons allow the positive, altruistic, act to proceed. Thus Step 4 is important because it enables us to evaluate the relative goodness of the act intended toward another person.

STEP 5: PERFORMANCE OF AN ALTRUISTIC ACT

The neurophysiology of motor control has occupied neuroscientists since the time of Nobel Prize–winning physiologist Sir Charles Sherrington, and is enlisted here to explain how a person carries out a beneficial act. The prosocial decision has occurred in Step 4. In Step 5 we leave the neuroscience that is specific to ABT and enter the common neuroscience of ordinary movement control. The output from the prefrontal cortex permits the motor cortex and subcortical movement-control neurons to perform the act that was so rapidly and automatically evaluated. In our 9/11 example, Siller swings into action, forgoes the day off with his brothers, and heads for the Tunnel to try and save other lives. He proceeds because he envisions himself in the target person's place. Any one of the generic "persons" that he imagines in the tower is sufficient to motivate his altruistic act. Step 5 is necessary to turn an ethical decision by neurons in the frontal cortex into an actual behavior. The positive, generous act occurs because it matches the way he himself would wish to be treated.

In summary, through the series of five ABT steps the brain carries out the neurohormonal mechanisms that produce behavior obeying an ethical universal, commonly called the Golden Rule. It should be emphasized here that such behavior is not part of a "bargain," where one person does something nice for another (because she thinks that the other will do something nice for her), and then that other reciprocates (out of obligation). The brain mechanisms just described do not involve such calculation. They do not involve religious training or social conditioning. Rather they are precipitated because humans are wired to be altruistic. And, of course, that includes *reciprocal* altruism. Here's an illustration. Not long before I sat down to write this chapter, I was standing on a subway platform when an old man emerged from a train pushing a cart full of groceries. When he got to the stairs leading to the exit, he stopped, wondering how he would possibly drag that cart up. But just then, a young man who was about to enter the train said "Wait, I'll do that for you," and he pulled the cart up to the top of the stairs. By the time he returned to the platform, he had missed his train, and I asked him in my best field-study voice "Why did you do that?" Acting genuinely surprised, he replied "Why wouldn't I? I just did what I had to." Indeed. Though he would never see that other man again, he felt the natural urge to help someone who could not help himself. He did this even though he would miss his train. The point is that he didn't stop to calculate whether to put someone else's needs ahead of his own.

So now let's explore still further reaches of ABT.

AVOIDANCE OF ANTISOCIAL BEHAVIOR

Because ABT deals with two classes of behavior (the first type being altruistic/good), let's now deal with the second type, that is, when we avoid doing something bad. Here a person's brain makes a decision to refrain from carrying out a nasty act against another person, let's say the murder of a competitor in a jealous rage. Again, ABT posits that during the next few hundredths of a second, the potential murderer's brain will follow the same five key steps.

The first three steps (representation, perception, and merging of images) are exactly the same as for the altruistic act. The next two steps differ.

Step 4: The Altruistic Brain

Representation of the act (from Step 1) and the united, combined image (from Step 3) arrive at the "ethical switch" in the person's brain. If a potential killer, for example, was planning to murder another person, the combined self/other signal is sent to the prefrontal cortex. There, Altruistic Brain neurons *are unable to register the difference* between the effects on the target and on himself and they inhibit motor cortex neurons that might have carried out the heinous act. While this may occur at a conscious level, it also can be instantaneous and unconscious. Altruistic Brain mechanisms in the prefrontal cortex also, of course, inhibit nasty acts much less serious than murder. Mechanisms for this are spelled out in Chapter 3.

Step 5: Behavior. Decline to Perform an Antisocial Act

In this case, Altruistic Brain neurons in the prefrontal cortex prevent motor acts that would harm another person. No harmful act takes place.

As you can see, avoidance of the nasty act achieves the same result as performance of the altruistic act: benevolence. The first three steps in the Altruistic Brain program are, in fact, identical in both scenarios. Step 4 differs because in the avoidance scenario the potential bad actor is revolted by the consequences of what he could do, whereas in the altruistic scenario he feels the glow of satisfaction. Step 5 is also different. The potential killer declines to perform the harmful act in the avoidance scenario, but in its altruistic counterpart he willingly performs the altruistic act.

This "avoidance" scenario, like its "performance" counterpart, is also totally spontaneous in the sense that humans are wired to produce good (and avoid bad) behavior. I am reminded of when one of my friends was furious at her neighbor whose dogs never stopped barking. She and the neighbor got into regular shouting matches. She wanted to push the woman and make her physically suffer. But did she? "No," she said, "something always restrained me." Of course, we can all identify with such restraint, which represents ABT in action. If community is built on being kind to others, it also relies on not doing things that hurt. It is this combination of action and restraint that is part of our evolutionary equipment, and that has contributed so profoundly to our species' survival.

A Parsimonious Theory

Scientists call a theory "elegant" when it efficiently explains a lot of phenomena without making a lot of special assumptions. Steps 1 through 5 do not require the brain to have any special "religious" capacities or any superhuman discriminatory powers. In fact, information is *lost* by the merging of images that occurs in Step 3.

So think about these scenarios of performing prosocial behaviors and avoiding antisocial behaviors for a moment, both positively altruistic and that based on avoidance. Nothing in either requires the brain to do anything extraordinary. ABT is plausible because all of the mechanisms on which it relies are (as the next chapter shows) well understood. Each step that it posits has its counterpart in fundamental experiments that have shown them to work. There is no supposition involved. The theory establishes that these steps can operate together, programmatically, and that when they do a person will behave in a manner that is altruistic. So what will really matter in the next phase of our journey, now that we have briefly reviewed the five steps of ABT, will be to visit some neuroscience labs where we can examine work that proves that Altruistic actions rely on trains of physiological events that include mundane sensory-motor data.

But to make the chapter's main point using different terms, ABT demonstrates that an ethical decision by one person about to act toward another involves only the *loss* of information, which is all too easy to achieve, as anyone who just forgot something will tell you. I reemphasize that the theory does not require special abilities. Indeed, learning complex information and storing it in memory are hard to explain. On the other hand, damping or suppressing any one of the many mechanisms involved in perception and memory are easy to achieve and can explain the blurring of identity required by this explanation of altruistic behavior. In the "potential murder" example imagined earlier, a loss of individuality as a result of blurred identity temporarily puts the potential murderer in the other person's place. Because that other person would be afraid, so will the potential actor. He avoids an unethical act because of shared fear.

All of the findings summarized in this chapter demonstrate how our brains can do the job of producing altruistic behaviors. Most important, several independent mechanisms allow image-of-other to blend with image-of-self, to foster the production of altruistic behaviors. These mechanisms are not exclusive of each other—they could work in various combinations—and those combinations could be different among different individuals.

Sometimes generous people contribute to causes, their behavior not seeming to reflect altruism toward an individual but rather toward an abstract entity. I conjecture that in all such cases the generous person has the "idea" of a person in mind. That is, she brings to mind a vision of that person. If the idea is generosity toward a library, then the generous person imagines a librarian. If it is brave acts in a crippled Japanese nuclear power plant, then the altruistic person imagines the image of a Fukushima villager. ABT, exactly as presented here, would apply.

APPLICATION OF ABT TO REAL-LIFE SITUATIONS

Having explained the five steps essential to ABT—steps that use ordinary brain mechanisms that neuroscientists work with every day—I now want to weave these steps into stories of good human behavior ranging from the smallest to the most serious examples. My point will be to illustrate how ABT actually plays out, how the individual steps can actually be mapped onto human acts. Thus though we cannot see the brain during the few hundredths of a second that it takes to make an altruistic decision, we can nonetheless identify how the brain is working as that decision is formulated and carried out.

Kindness

It was one of those days when the sun's glare off shadeless streets made everyone wince. I was just beginning to cross Third Avenue in Manhattan when I saw that a limousine had stalled. The overweight, middle-aged driver was breaking into an impressive sweat, straining to push his vehicle out of the traffic and into a parking space on East 65th Street. Just then, a slim, smartly dressed young man changed his direction and approached. It was obvious that he didn't know the driver, and was under no obligation to offer a hand and mess up his pristine suit in the process. Yet when I looked back, he had put down his expensive-looking briefcase and was pushing the stalled limo to a safe spot. Why?

I never got a chance to ask him, but his spontaneous action was of a piece with the heroics of Wesley Autrey, albeit on a much smaller scale. Think about ABT's five steps. (Step 1) The young man's brain represented the limousine-pushing action. Neurons that would have to direct the straining and stressful movements caused by contraction of the driver's leg and back muscles send corollary discharges to the young man's sensory systems. (Step 2) The young man's visual cortex got the electrical signals of neurons representing the visual image of the overweight driver, and (Step 3) merged the driver's visual image with his own, using one or more of the mechanisms I introduced in Step Three above. Sent to the prefrontal cortex, this combination signaled to Altruistic Brain neurons there (Step 4) obviously resulted in a sense of relief from help pushing the limousine and these prefrontal neurons told motor cortex neurons "Yes," "Do It." As a result (Step 5) the young man pushed the limo to a safe spot using his own motor control systems, both cortical and subcortical.

Though this action would not be considered heroic, it constitutes one of the myriad kindnesses that we perform literally without thinking. In any given instance, we do not even calculate whether someone will sometime help us, as kindnesses are unconsciously traded all day long in a kind of unregulated moral economy. We go through life giving each other a hand, running down the Up escalator to retrieve someone's dropped glove. It's this low-level back-and-forth of kindness that makes life tolerable, that we think about after the fact as opposed to in advance. Evidence of ABT is everywhere. It gives us reassurance and, indeed, a measure of courage in the face of adversity.

Everyday Heroes

When you start thinking about the everyday heroes around us, either in the neighborhood or on the news, there are so many: not just people who do good deeds, but those who flat out risk their lives (or even give them) without stopping to calculate the odds. For example, a few months after Wesley Autrey startled the world, another less celebrated hero saved even more young people. This was Professor Liviu Librescu, a Holocaust survivor who taught engineering at Virginia Tech. When a deranged student, Seung-Hui Cho, started rampaging through campus—finally killing 32 and wounding 17—Librescu blocked his classroom door with his own body, giving students the chance to escape. While most made it out the windows to safety, Librescu never emerged alive, taking several bullets through the door. His family was in shock, but his son told an Israeli newspaper that people said "my father was a hero." And there have been others.

In July, 2012, a horrific drama played out where a group of young people, at the expense of their own lives, saved loved ones from a deranged gunman. At a premier of *Batman: The Dark Knight Rises*, James McQuinn, 27, threw his body in front of his girlfriend and took two bullets meant for her. Jonathan Blunk, 26, a military veteran, also died when he saved his girlfriend. How did they so react so courageously?

Think about this as instantaneous, unconscious applications of ABT in action. These two young men (Step 1) had in their brains the "corollary discharge" representation of their movements, to throw themselves protectively in front of their girlfriends, and obviously (Step 2) had the visual images of these women merged with their own (Step 3). These motor and sensory neural signals sent (Step 4) to Altruistic Brain mechanisms in the prefrontal cortex rapidly and emotionally yielded a "Go," "Do it" decision because of the positive valence associated with saving the two women's lives. As a result (Step 5) they leapt, thus performing the ultimate prosocial act. They didn't stop to think whether the other person was "worth it," or whether the odds were in favor of their personal survival. They just acted. Because we have seen this type of action involving total strangers, we know that the motivating factor was not—in some soap-opera sense— undying love. We know that neurohormonal processes kicked in at lightning speed, changing some people's lives forever. Ultimately, the community benefits from this type of action, which is why—in evolutionary terms—we can have expected it. Those who expressed surprise and admiration should have shelved their surprise and admired the human brain.

Earthquake, Tsunami, Meltdown

The whole world felt like an unintended and infernal field study when in March, 2011, a continuous loop of coverage depicted the Japanese earthquake, the tsunami that followed, and finally the flooded Fukushima nuclear plant that contaminated an area the size of New Jersey. In the ensuing days, as the magnitude of the tragedy—and the danger—became apparent, people from all over Japan volunteered to clean up the environment and stabilize the plant. Their narratives form a mosaic of unfettered selflessness, a commitment to their fellow citizens that held the world in thrall. CNN, for example, reported a story with the title "Japanese seniors volunteer for Fukushima 'suicide corps,'" about hundreds of older people willing to don emergency gear so that they could work inside the crippled plant. One such man, however, Masaaki Takahashi, 65, said that he didn't understand all the fuss over their efforts. "I want them to stop calling us the 'suicide corps' or kamikazes. We're doing nothing special. I simply think I have to do something and I can't allow just young people to do this." One hears Wesley Autrey ("You should do the right thing") in this quiet acceptance of a moral code impelling him to act on behalf of others. Another member of the group, Kazuko Sasaki, 69, articulated a sense of responsibility that he also could not ignore: "My generation, the older generation, promoted the nuclear plants. If we don't take responsibility, who will?" (Figure 2-2).

And consider an *ABC News* story entitled "Japan's Fukushima 50: Heroes who volunteered to stay behind at Japan's Crippled Nuclear Plants." The "50" were actually 200 seasoned technicians, who worked in shifts of 50 so as to avoid the worst doses of radiation through prolonged exposure. But their conditions were still almost unendurable. According to the story "They are working as temperatures at the plants soar to nerve wracking levels, radiation is leaking, rain may be carrying it down upon them, and a toxic fire burns, likely spewing more radiation into the

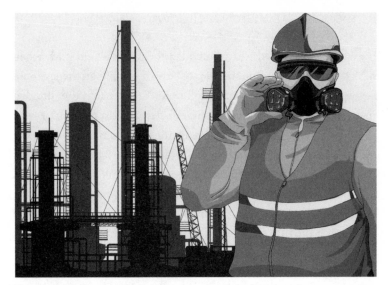

Figure 2.2 Following the explosion at the Fukushima nuclear power plant, Japanese workers exposed themselves to danger in order to cool the plant down and prevent greater risks to the population in northern Japan.

atmosphere.... They've gone into battle, crawling at times through dark mazes, armed with flashlights and radiation detectors, wearing full body hazmat suits and breathing through cumbersome oxygen tanks." What's fascinating is that these were ordinary men who rose to the occasion. In a tweet picked up by several news services, one woman said of her neighbor: "At home, he doesn't seem like someone who could handle big jobs... but today I was really proud of him." The hazards faced by the Fukushima 50 were big news. The *New York Times* reported:

> Those [workers] remaining are being asked to make escalat-ing —and perhaps existential—sacrifices—that so far are only being implicitly acknowledged.
>
> Japan's Health Ministry said Tuesday it was raising the legal limit on the amount of radiation to which each worker could be

exposed, to 250 millisieverts from 100 millisieverts, five times the maximum exposure permitted for American nuclear plants.

Nonetheless, the workers kept rotating in and out of the plant, with apparently none giving up. It was observed that "Nuclear reactor operators say that their profession is typified by the same kind of esprit de corps found among fire fighters and elite military units." This commitment, both to one another and to society, was borne out in an email from the daughter of one of the 50: "He says he's accepted his fate ... much like a death sentence." Less dramatically, but with no less certitude, an American consultant, Michael Friedlander, observed: "I can tell you with 100 percent certainty they are absolutely committed to doing whatever is humanly necessary to make these plants [stabilized] in safe condition, even at the risk of their own lives."

As the events unfolded, people in the street were too scared to psychoanalyze the 50. One such person, Maeda Akihiro, said: "They're putting their life on the line. If that place blows up, it's the end for all of us, so all I can do is send them encouragement." But as I will argue, the individual psychologies of these men—where they grew up, whether they had served in Japan's armed forces—was never the critical issue. Rather, the men exemplified a common human capacity to act in the interest of others, even in the face of danger. Of course, this is not to diminish their heroism in the slightest, but only to suggest how they made their decision to act and how they remained committed to it. The Fukushima disaster will be studied for years by planners hoping to prevent another such occurrence, but if there is one positive side to the story it is that human beings acted so well. It was one example among many.

Now think of the decision that an individual Fukushima worker had to make in terms of the five steps of ABT. (Step 1) He represents in his own brain the action of re-entering the nuclear plant to cool it and prevent an explosion. From his premotor cortex, signals emanate that yield the corollary discharge that informs his own sensory systems of what he is about to do. (Step 2) He envisions the generic farmer and village dweller in the Fukushima area. This envisioning uses standard visual signaling pathways. (Step 3) Losing the distinction between his self-image and that of the local Fukushima citizen, by the three mechanisms I introduced previously and will explain in Chapter 3, he literally "identifies with" that citizen in his cerebral cortex. (Step 4) Signals of the explosion-preventing act combined with his self/citizen merged image reach Altruistic Brain neurons in the prefrontal cortex, leading to a "Yes," "this is good." (Step 5) The Fukushima worker reenters the plant. No secondary explosions occur.

We could go on studying examples of outstandingly altruistic behavior such as that by Oskar Schindler, who saved Jewish citizens from the Holocaust; Doctors Without Borders (Medecins Sans Frontières), an international medical humanitarian organization created in France; and kidney and bone marrow donors across the country. However, I have already made the point: exemplary behavior can be understood at the level of basic brain research.

Neuroscientific Evidence

Now that I have provided a brief outline of how ABT explains the decision to act in an ethical, even altruistic fashion, Chapter 3 will open up the neuroscience laboratory to allow you to appreciate some of the vast scientific evidence for how such behavior is activated. I will now share some of this thrill with you, so that you can see how the pieces (or rather, steps) of ABT fall into place. And then, beyond the ethical decision, we'll look at why we actually behave in an altruistic way: both neuronal and hormonal forces that have evolved among vertebrate animals will provide the "drive" to accomplish the deed. Consider this automotive analogy: if the Altruistic Brain turns the switch so that the engine is on, these neuronal and hormonal forces provide the fuel for the engine to move the car forward. Chapter 4 talks about these forces as well.

FURTHER READING

Katherine Cullen. 2004. "Sensory Signals During Active versus Passive Movement." *Current Opinion in Neurobiology* 14, 698–706.

Anthony Damasio. 2010. *Self Comes to Mind*. New York: Pantheon.

Richard Held and Sanford Freedman. 1963. "Plasticity in Human Sensorimotor Control. *Science* 142, 455–462.

H. Lau, Robert D. Rogers, Patrick Haggard, and Richard E. Passingham. 2004. "Attention to Intention." *Science* 303, 1208–1211.

[3]

PRIMARY NEUROSCIENCE RESEARCH UNDERLYING EACH STEP OF ALTRUISTIC BRAIN THEORY

Each step of the Altruistic Brain Theory (ABT) is grounded in primary research, reported in the literature of neuroscience. By "literature" scientists mean a type of report that not only describes an experimental result according to strict scientific standards, but is also vetted by and published in the world's peer-reviewed journals. These results are then tested and confirmed by further such reports. By the time a result appears in the literature and receives imprimatur in still further studies, it is considered part of scientists' common knowledge, reliable enough to serve as the basis for their ongoing research.

So now let's take the steps one by one, examining in each case how they are supported by specific studies.

NEURAL BASIS OF STEP 1: HOW WE CAN REPRESENT AN ACT IN OUR BRAIN BEFORE UNDERTAKING THAT ACT

Many lines of evidence show that we represent an action to ourselves before we actually undertake it. The simplest type of study, a representation far less complex than one involving altruistic behavior, involves eye–hand coordination. In this instance, the evidence involves eye movement, one of the best examples of how the brain previews its upcoming action. Consider this: when a person turns his eyes to the right, does his visual world appear to jump to the left? No. Nor is the visual signal deranged by the eye movement. The person's visual scene remains stable because the motor command for the eye movement *is represented to the rest of this person's brain* slightly before it actually happens, and so the person's brain, as a result, has already corrected for the eye movement (see Figure 3-1). This type of demonstration and hundreds of other studies show that representation of one's body movement in one's own brain has been important in neurophysiological research for a long time.

I have worked in the tradition started by scientists whom you might call "engineers-turned-psychologists." Their experiments were the first to explore a neurophysiological phenomenon called "corollary discharge," which refers to the extra motor signals that are sent over to the sensory pathways to notify the sensory pathways that the world will appear to change as a result of the movement. Studies of corollary discharge proved an idea—"reafferenz"—originated by German engineer/psychologists. "Reafferenz" meant that just prior to and during movement our nervous system not only gets its regular sensory ("afferent") input but also gets notice ("reafferent") of the movements we are about to make.

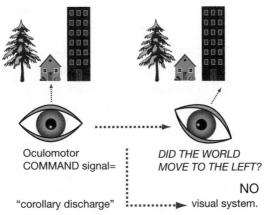

Figure 3.1 When we move our eyes to the right, does the world appear to jump to the left? No. This is because the same motor neurons that tell the eye muscles what to do also represent that movement to the visual system so that the visual system expects such an eye movement. "Corollary discharge" means the common phenomenon that the brain represents intended movements to its appropriate sensory systems.

Here is how it works. "Representing our impending actions to ourselves" does not mean that we consciously observe a little play in which we are performing. Everything happens rapidly, automatically, and in most cases unconsciously. A long history of neurophysiological work tells us that actions we are about to take are represented to our own brains. In some cases that scientific work also makes clear why this occurs. Almost 50 years ago, Erich von Holst asked why, if a person's body is moving, his world does not just spin. He theorized that every movement is signaled to the individual's central nervous system, and then is compared to the resulting change in visual angle so that the originator of the movement can distinguish between the effect of his own movement and an actual change in the angle of visually perceived objects.

Scientists at Brandeis and MIT have performed experiments to study the necessity for active movements in our visual and auditory environments, movements represented to our own brains to maintain our sense of stability. Most telling were those in which volunteers were asked to wear prisms over their eyes. The prisms changed the apparent visual angle in the volunteers' visual field by, for example, 30 degrees. When a volunteer would reach for an object his reach would be misdirected by the corresponding angle, 30 degrees. Only if he was allowed to make active movements with the prisms on, with those movements and their consequences relayed back to his brain, was he able to compensate for the prisms and reach toward the object accurately: the brain kept track. It is subliminally and instantly aware of actions and their consequences. These active movements and the signals emanating from them are crucial for normal eye–hand coordination.

I showed that the same principle applies to hearing, working with colleagues Sanford Friedman and engineer/psychologist Richard Held. When the loudness and timing of sounds reaching our left and right ears change with regard to the balance between left and right, is that because we are moving or because the source of the sound is moving? It is because the representation of our own movement while we make it allows us to keep track. Moreover, suppose that we start to lift something of indeterminate weight. The comparison between the force that our muscles exert and the sensory feedback from them tells us how much more force we must use to lift the weight at a given speed or to a given height. All of these examples derive from the neurophysiology of ordinary motor control.

All of this scientific detail concerning simple sensory-motor coordination demonstrates that the first step of ABT, in which one represents one's impending action to oneself in one's own brain, is business-as-usual, an accepted neurophysiological fact.

Indeed, the brain's ability to anticipate its own motor commands uses the same neuronal capacity that we use when we anticipate actions toward another person. As already explained, when the motor control systems in our brains send previewing signals of impending acts over to the sensory systems, called corollary discharges because they are a simple consequence of the main motor command signal. The most prominent scientist currently exploring the field of corollary discharge is McGill University neurophysiologist Katherine Cullen. Cullen states that in all vertebrates—humans, monkeys, fish, and all other animals with backbones—the central nervous system keeps track of where we are and where we are going, so as to monitor our relation to the world. In fact, Cullen suggests, "this ability is essential for perceptual stability as well as accurate motor control." She has shown that cells in our lower brainstem compare actual body position to signals calculated from desired and expected body position. When desired actual body positions are identical to each other, the motion needed to accomplish the expected body position is complete. In recent experiments, Michael Goldberg at Columbia has discovered neurons, in the part of the brain that deals with vision, where neuronal activities anticipate movements. Such discoveries of mundane motor acts regulated by presignaling demonstrate that the first step of the altruistic brain theory is ordinary, as we always represent an impending action to ourselves.

That the brain anticipates and logs its impending actions has also emerged with regard to other parts of the nervous system, not just the motor cortex. In a part of the forebrain essential for our awareness of ourselves, the midline thalamus, nerve cell activities reveal that we depend on premotor signals of our eyes and other parts of our bodies to guide all physical actions. Scientists have extensively characterized these neurons in the thalamus of monkeys, and found that such cells were active during eye movements and that firing patterns could precede eye positioning. They then discovered that there were at least two kinds of such cells: those responding to a visual stimulus transiently, to detect a stimulus toward which the eyes should move; and other neurons with sustained responses that could provide a signal holding the monkey's gaze upon the target. Thus, as became apparent in the later results, not all thalamic neurons keeping track of eye movements are the same. Variations across this nerve cell population in the exact timing of electrical activity associated with rapid eye movements suggest a variety of ways in which this function is served. The thalamic neurons that keep track of our eye movements would seem to be important for our ability to orient correctly toward a visual stimulus.

Of course, viewed in isolation all of these neurophysiological studies may appear quite remote from moral behavior. But they also demonstrate the total pervasiveness of presignaling motor commands in the brain—a crucial step in ABT. Nor is this type of presignaling limited to higher animals and humans. Electrophysiological experiments with singing crickets, carried out recently in Switzerland, narrowed the cellular basis for these copies of our motor signals down to a single type of neuron. In this simple animal, a powerful neuron, neither purely sensory nor purely motor, coordinated activities of several parts of the body and mediated the animal's ability to keep track of its own action.

At this point, it should be clear that a very large number of lines of evidence support Step 1 of the ABT, and that we (along with other creatures) regularly represent anticipated actions to ourselves before we actually perform them. It seems to be a widespread natural strategy for coping with the world. As the neurologist Antonio Damasio says in *Self Comes to Mind*, "the business of managing life consists of managing a body and the management gains precision and efficiency from the presence of a brain." Communications between brain and body go both ways, from body to brain, and from brain to body. So if managing the living body is our main job, then "brain mapping (of signals from the body) is the enabler, the engine that transforms plain life regulation into minded regulation."

All of this neurophysiological and behavioral evidence shows that there is nothing mysterious about the brain's ability to represent movements. A brain *must* represent its actions to itself in order to keep track of the relation between those action and their consequences. That is how it maintains stability in a changing world. While ABT depends on this ability, the neural mechanisms involved are in no way limited to ethics or special to ethical behavior. They are, rather, part of a well-established neurophysiological design that spans many species.

NEURAL BASIS OF STEP 2: HOW WE CAN PERCEIVE THE TARGET OF AN INTENDED ACT

How does one perceive the person toward whom one intends to act? Not easily. The great advances in the neuroscience of vision during the second half of the 20th century dealt with visually simple stimuli such as individual lines at particular angles. These discoveries were made by recording from individual neurons in the primary visual cortex, the part of our cerebral cortex that receives visual signals directly from the thalamus. At the same time, we knew that some mechanisms special for perceiving faces would emerge sooner or later because the great neurologists had, in the late 19th century, found difficulties in face perception after damage to the cortex. How do we see the intended target of our action if she is right in front of us?

When we see this other person, this visual information is processed by our brains so that an image of that person is virtually "constructed" in the brain. The question is: how does this happen? Consider perception of a face as the paradigm of how we perceive another person. The very first discoveries, in the 1970s, were made by Charles Gross at Princeton, who began to find startling properties of cells in an area of the cortex that he had been studying for a long time, an area far removed from the primary visual cortex. While the primary visual cortex is at the very back of the brain, Charlie's recorded neurons are farther forward and to the side, in a region called inferotemporal cortex. Most important in relation to Step 2, he discovered neurons that would respond only to faces. Some neurons responded best to faces shown in profile; others responded to frontal views of the faces. Though these electrical recordings were obtained from nerve cells in monkey brains, it is obvious that similar mechanisms operate in the human brain. In neuroanatomical work that confirmed and extended Gross' electrophysiology, MIT Professor Nancy Kanwisher used functional magnetic resonance imaging (fMRI) and found a convincing "face recognition module" in one part of the human brain. She even identified specific electromagnetic waves associated with the categorization of visual stimuli as faces and the successful recognition of individual faces.

For a long time, neuroscientists had supposed that our ability to see other people would depend on what they jokingly called "grandmother cells"—neurons that would fire only if the image of our grandmother (i.e., someone who, in general, we would recognize) passed in front of our eyes and therefore allowed us to recognize her. However, we now understand that there are sets of face-selective neurons that are actually members of large ensembles of neurons for recognizing faces. Indeed, Japanese scientists found individual nerve cells that respond only to particular features of the face or head. From their results, we know that facial recognition can depend on patterns of activity among populations of cortical neurons. This is more complex than the idea of "grandmother neurons."

What about the case when the beneficiary is not right in front of the person who is going to perform an altruistic act, but instead exists as a generic "image"—for example, as a wounded person in the Twin Towers? In such a situation, the visual representation of that generic person must be there, in the cortex, but neuroscience does not yet know how that envisioning process is initiated.

In summary, we all want our percepts—our sensory signals—to be clear and accurate, a neurophysiological challenge. ABT posits the opposite, the nonchallenging case in which our sensory signals are unclear—as Step 3 explains.

NEURAL BASIS OF STEP 3: HOW IMAGES OF ACTOR AND TARGET CAN MERGE IN THE BRAIN

What does it mean to "merge images?" For Step 3 of ABT, suppose that the visual signal from the target of one's intended action is signaled by cortical neurons, as Step 2 explained. But for the brain to direct moral behavior, visual images will *not* remain separate, clear, and individually distinct. Instead, an image of the face of the person toward whom one will act is blurred with the image of oneself. Because visual perception is so difficult to perfect, as you can imagine from Step 2, you can understand how easy it is to reduce precision of the visual imaging of faces. Saying that facial images must be "merged" means that when nerve cells are activated and signal the other person's face, they excite the neurons whose activity will signal one's own self-image. This process is called "cross-excitation."

First, let's consider how this process is even possible. After all, we tend to think of the brain as literally translating objects in the world into images that more or less correspond to those objects, and retain a degree of integrity that allows us to see these objects as both whole and discrete. Yet, as I am about to explain, there are many occasions when this does not happen, so that what actually registers in the brain—that is, what we actually "see"—is not a literal translation from what exists in the world. Once I have established that this is so, I will explain the detailed cellular mechanisms underlying the merger of images.

To satisfy the theory, we must be able to "see the other person as ourselves." For example, nerve cell signaling that represents the face of the person toward whom we will act must be channeled into the nerve cell pathways that represent our own face's self-image. But how would face signals emanating from the face of our action's target merge into the signals from our own face? This is the central question, going to the heart of ABT. The brain can easily join two images together—reduce the precision of visual signaling—in any part of the multistaged set of mechanisms by which visual information reaches the primary visual cortex and then gets transmitted to a subsequent, more sophisticated part of the cortex. This reduction of precision offers the opportunity to join our own image with the image of the object of our intended actions.

Here is one way to understand how the merging or joining of images can take place. It has to do with "cell assemblies," groups of neurons that enable us to recognize faces. If any one part of a cell assembly is turned off, the function of that cell assembly is not accomplished. It is easy to make a cell assembly *not* function, by altering the chemistry of one of those cells in the assembly or by altering their hookups. Thus if cells are not working in the relevant part of the cerebral cortex, a special part of the temporal lobe of the cerebral cortex essential for face recognition, that would reduce our ability to recognize and think about a person's individual visual image, and correspondingly increase the opportunity to see the other person's image as our own. As a consequence, using the mechanisms spelled out later, the *lack* of precision of facial perception can be achieved as required by ABT.

Detailed neuroscience discoveries support the idea that reduction of face perception is easy to accomplish. In the first place, face-selective regions are located primarily in the right side of the cerebral cortex, not the left, so we do not have left–right redundancy to maintain individual face recognition. Moreover, as Kanwisher pointed out to me, simply adding electrical noise—random, confusing little signals—in the electrical signaling among neurons in the cortex, or altering slightly the timing and phasing of arrival of facial information at the cortex, would *reduce discriminability* among faces. This is easy. All neurophysiologists know that "noise" in neural systems is easy to come by, and by reducing discriminability among faces it serves the function of ABT.

One of the greatest features of the human brain is its great ability to take in and process visual signals. But ABT mechanisms generalize to other senses—they work in the auditory realm as well. Even in the human brain, so dominated by visual systems, the sense of self need not be limited to *envisioning* oneself. For Antonio Damasio, writing in *Descartes' Error,* self-awareness depends on "numerous brain systems that must be in full swing." These would include "representations of our musculoskeletal frame and its potential movement," reconstructed on a moment-by-moment basis. An extension from Damasio could then include that facial recognition is also part of self-awareness and thus relevant to the explanation at hand. Several recent fMRI studies have pictured wide-ranging circuits in the human cerebral cortex that are activated by recognizing one's own face compared to others. But this applies as well to the feeling of being touched. For our purposes, the most important implication of these multiple and complex circuits is their susceptibility to blurring and confusion, easily achieved by the mechanisms highlighted in the next paragraph. Damping down, or suppressing any part of them, would allow us to run our sense of self together with that of another human being, as theorized in Step 3.

"Damping down" the difference between self and other operates by means that we can all recognize as feasible and easy to imagine. Think of any complex device, for example, the high-speed copier in your office. Is it easier to cause a breakdown or to repair it? Obviously, it is easier to reduce the performance of an office machine than it is to sustain it at peak efficiency. Indeed, it is hard to keep *any* complex device operating, but simple to reduce its performance by "throwing sand in the gears." Even small changes in a computer or TV hookup can undermine its performance dramatically. Therefore, it is clearly plausible to propose a reduction in operational efficiency of neural circuits that discriminate between oneself and "not-self," that is, another person. Think back to the sophisticated mechanisms detailed in Step 2. Reduced performance of *any* of those cerebral cortical circuits and mechanisms would blur individual identities. ABT says that to behave altruistically we simply *reduce* the precision of information transfer in the brain. That is easy.

One could, for example, depict an act to be avoided. A young man might be angry and intend to push someone in front of a bus. But during the interval, his mental image of the would-be target merges with his own. He is left with an instantaneous image of himself being pushed in front of the bus. Hence he desists.

The same scenario holds for a positive act toward the other person. For such a merging of images to happen here I describe specific, well-researched neuronal mechanisms that make Step 3 possible. That is, whereas previous paragraphs explained that the merger of images is theoretically possible under an array of different conditions, I now show how the brain actually does it and why we know this to be so.

There are well-established neural mechanisms for image merging. It is important to understand exactly how the brain achieves cross-excitation among images. Reduction and merging of images take place in the cerebral cortex by making the relevant neurons excitable enough that cross-excitation can occur. Cellular mechanisms to support such overexcitability are already known—following the next paragraph, I will provide not just one, but three detailed possible mechanisms for doing this. Each example is well established, and indeed could operate in parallel. Nor are they mutually exclusive and they could actually work in various combinations in different individuals.

But first, to understand cross-excitation, put yourself in the position of an "engineer" designing how the cerebral cortex will work as it becomes part of the human brain. As this imagined engineer, how do you design for cross-excitation among visual images?

a. *One way of merging images of two persons is to reduce the effectiveness of "inhibitory synapses" in the cortex.* A well-established, even classical feature of neural circuitry, the inhibitory synapse is a connection between nerve cells that causes the second cell to fire less. For example, the neurotransmitter gamma-aminobutyric acid (GABA) turns off electrical excitability in the nerve cells on which it impinges via "inhibitory synapses." Thus, one mechanism to increase nerve cell firing and cross-excitation among images would entail the *loss* of synaptic inhibition (Figure 3.2).

b. *Another way is to merge personal images by revving up the widespread excitatory inputs delivering the neurotransmitter*

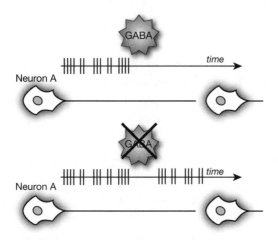

Figure 3.2 At the top, the GABA neuron that releases the inhibitory chemical GABA stops the signaling of neuron A. If the GABA-caused inhibition is reduced or eliminated, neuron A's excitation and signaling continues at a high rate. That is, with this loss of GABA inhibition happening in the cerebral cortex, cross-excitation between images—merging of images—results.

acetylcholine (ACh). This second, well-established mechanism entails increased excitation from the arousal neurotransmitter, ACh. ACh, a classically established and rather simple chemical, is known to be released from presynaptic endings and to turn on electrical activity in the postsynaptic neuron. Studies using electrical recording from neurons in the visual cortex, which were carried out specifically to look at the effects of ACh, showed massive electrophysiological effects. ACh enhances cognitive function and is an important influence on the overall arousal state of the cerebral cortex. Even small differences in the amount of ACh released in the cortex and the exact location of its release could greatly affect the *spread of excitation* between images of two people, actor and target. Thus, this step of ABT—the merging of another's image with self-image—is easily achieved through this mechanism involving increased ACh release.

c. *A third way is to increase cross-excitation among personal images by opening tiny tunnels, "gap junctions," between sensory cortical nerve cells, leading to widespread excitatory merging of two images.* This type of mechanism involves the rapid spread of excitation within a region of cerebral cortex owing to the operation of gap junctions (see Figure 3-3). Discovered in the 1980s and the subject of hundreds of scientific papers since then, these junctions allow a direct spread of electrical current from one nerve cell to another. Importantly, it is much easier for one cell to excite another through a gap junction than it is through a synapse; electrically charged atoms simply flood through the gap junction from one neuron to the next. Therefore, if images are to merge in the cerebral cortex, then rapid spread of excitation through gap junctions obviously helps to complete this step of ABT.

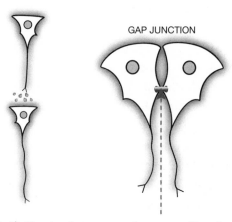

Figure 3.3 (Left) Sketch of conventional synapse. "Droplets" signify neurotransmitter. (Right) Gap junction allows rapid spread of electrical excitation from nerve cell to nerve cell, e.g., to merge images.

It is important to understand that all three of these theoretical mechanisms either collectively, separately, or in combination lead to high degrees of neuronal excitation, a spread of neuronal excitation that leads to a "cross-excitation" from one person's image to another. Because an image is composed of numerous lines, angles, and curves, the effective blurring of one image into another could be achieved simply by rendering the facial representations in the cerebral cortex from the other person to oneself more similar to each other, from line to line, angle to angle, and curve to curve. All three mechanisms provide for a merging of the image of the target of one's action to the image of the actor. And all three mechanisms could work in parallel, and different mechanisms could be most prominent in the brains of different people.

Even beyond cross-excitation between images, there are more opportunities to blend the image of the target of one's intended action with one's own image. We have so far established that partially reducing the efficiency of facial recognition pathways in the cerebral cortex would reduce individual face recognition and theoretically promote the sequence of steps that predispose us to treat others as ourselves. Moreover, because facial recognition mechanisms must be complex, this reduction of efficiency of face recognition pathways should be easy to accomplish; therefore it should be easy to explain how we behave as well as we do.

Additional ways of describing how facial percepts could blend into one another add strength to this theory. For example, consider the logic of so-called "whole/part relationships." For purposes of Step 3 of the ABT, that would mean the difference between "that is a face" (the whole) and "that is the individual face I recognize as my partner" (the part). The "whole" of whole/part, that is, generic face recognition, would allow a person to treat everyone as himself. Experiments by Charles Gilbert at Rockefeller University during electrical recordings from the cerebral cortex of an experimental animal emphasize the flexibility with which visual objects can be grouped by the perceiver. Thus, Gilbert's result further satisfies Step 3 by allowing us flexibly to render any face of the person toward whom we'd be acting together with our own self-image.

This notion of "whole/part relations" gained powerful support when I approached my Rockefeller University colleague, neurophysiologist Winrich Freiwald, who records from neurons in the cerebral cortex so as to crack the face recognition problem. I broached the ideas that I am discussing now, and asked for his insights. Specifically, when I asked "what might be the mechanisms that would most easily blend different facial images so that they would seem very similar?" he responded, "Don, there are at least two components to your question. One is that face recognition starts with face detection. You've got to know that there is *a face* out there. The second component is face categorization, including individuation among faces. Interestingly, we found lots of cells in the most anterior group of face recognition cells that *were invariant to identity*. It does still amaze me that this is the case, but it might reflect the need to have a representation of a general face." Another independent answer to the problem—how images of others could be likened to images of ourselves for the purpose of guiding social behavior—may have arisen a few meters from my lab: cortical nerve cells whose responses tend to minimize differences among different faces.

Supporting Winrich's detailed nerve cell by nerve cell recordings, neuroscientists have recently recorded brain waves from large numbers of patients' brains. They report electrical responses to the images of faces that are absent when other visual stimuli, such as strings of letters, are flashed in front of the patients' eyes. Most important, according to these electrical recording results in the human brain, there are "early stages" of face processing and "later stages" of face processing. ABT would say that those early stages likely indicate that "this is a human face." It could be my face or the face of the person toward whom I will act.

So-called "mirror neurons" help, as well. Step 3 gains still more support from another direction: cerebral cortical "mirror neurons." If the cortical neurons that minimize difference among faces could be thought of as scientific gifts from "brain research heaven," another entirely different gift was tossed over to New York from Italy. This was the discovery of neurons called "mirror cells." Mirror cells provide still another major mechanism for altruistic behavior. Some people think that "mirror cells," first studied in Italy several years ago, comprise the most important discovery in biology since DNA.

One morning in the Universita di Parma, in Italy, neurophysiologists in the laboratory of Giacomo Rizzolatti were recording from a nerve cell in an area of a monkey's cerebral cortex called the premotor cortex. This cell would fire action potentials when the monkey raised its right arm to a horizontal position. Then the scientists paused for lunch, across the room. They were startled, during lunch, to hear that nerve cell, still being recorded, firing vigorously. Why? It turned out that the monkey's premotor nerve cell would also fire when the monkey's brain saw an experimenter's right arm in that same horizontal position as when he held a cup of coffee during lunch. This part of the monkey's brain activity "identified with" the corresponding part of the experimenter's brain activity. Even more striking was their observation that in a different part of the monkey cortex, some neurons fired early enough during a temporal series of actions that Rizzolatti and his colleagues could conclude that "these neurons not only code the observed motor act but also allow the observer to understand the agent's intentions." Such neurons could easily form the basis of empathy. As such, these neurons are made to order for Step 3 of ABT because they would allow one person to put himself in another person's place.

The prestigious journal *Science* called Rizzolatti's discovery "the most interesting finding in biology since DNA." Mirror neurons are all the more interesting now that Rizzolatti's collaborator, Vittorio Gallese, has reported that evidence for such neurons can be found in the human brain as well. "If I have nerve cells in my brain that react the same way corresponding nerve cells react in your brain when you make a certain movement, then I am, almost literally, 'putting myself in your shoes.' Extending this, if I as a routine can put myself in your place, then the essential step of my empathizing with you is *automatically* accomplished!"

In Step 3 of the theory, all of the mechanisms cited above can work together or separately to guarantee the blurring of images between the image of the target person and that of the would-be actor's. Remember that all of these mechanisms for merging images in our brains could work in various combinations, and different combinations could be important in different individuals. This kind of flexibility and multiplicity of brain mechanisms leading to altruism—image-blurring—virtually guarantees that the brain can actually perform according to ABT.

To summarize Step 3, the loss of face-recognition information is an essential element of ABT. The recognition of another person depends on a long series of electrophysiological and biochemical reactions to the stimuli particular to that person. These include not only seeing the other person's face, but also hearing his voice, feeling his touch, and smelling his personal odors. Every one of our senses must work hard to identify someone as a particular person, who is not just anyone in general, and who is not oneself. Reduction of that ability to make such discriminations in any of these sensory pathways will result in a blurring of the target's identity. In such instances, a person is less easy to discriminate from others and, indeed, from oneself.

Consider the many mechanisms just discussed that could provide the essential blurring of identity. This plethora of different mechanisms makes it especially likely that one or another will actually work in the manner just illustrated. They all could work independently, and in fact different ones could be most important in different individuals. Precisely because there are so many ways for ABT to work, I believe that it accounts for the robust character of human prosocial behavior.

NEURAL BASIS OF STEP 4: WHEN THE BRAIN EVALUATES AN IMPENDING ACTION, THEN IT CAUSES A PROSOCIAL ACT

Thinking back to the example used in Chapter 2, Steven Siller's brain evaluates the intended action as to whether it will benefit or harm a World Trade Tower recipient. Step 4 unfolds when the positive or negative import for feelings and thus for action is determined. Siller's cortex will have to link the blurred image and intended action to parts of the brain that will evaluate what results they might lead to. Then the message, appropriately processed, will be headed for an emotionally loaded "ethical switch," a mechanism in the brain influenced by positive or negative emotional consequences. Steven Siller will feel good if he knows that (on account of his actions) a rescue will feel good; he will feel unhappy if he knows that the target of his heroic action would for some reason be unhappy. In both cases, an altruistic, prosocial act is precipitated.

I use the phrase "emotionally loaded" ethical switch because I am in the business of explaining the altruistic component of an ethical act, and emotions have always been a subject of ethical philosophy. Indeed, few people would fail to worry if a neighbor gets badly hurt or to be happy if that neighbor experienced good fortune. So in Step 4 the brain of our intrepid actor—Steven Siller—will combine the represented act (Step 1) and merged images (Steps 2 and 3) so as to evaluate the emotional consequences.

In Step 4, visual signals that identify individuals—as well as other such signals including sound, touch, and odor—are sent from the cortex to another part of the forebrain, the prefrontal cortex. As you will see from the studies of Joshua Greene's lab, discussed in Chapter 5, the most likely candidates for sites where these signals converge would be cells within the prefrontal cortex, based on its regulation of many forms of emotionally significant behavior. The amygdala would also be such a site because of its importance in the regulation of emotion. There is good precedent for sensory information connected with moral judgments being sent to areas of the brain traditionally connected with emotion. A binational team spanning the globe from Rome to Los Angeles used functional magnetic resonance imaging (fMRI) to track neuronal activity in specific parts of the brain, while the subject either imitated or simply observed facial expressions obviously reflecting emotion. They found greater neuronal activity during active imitation as compared to simply observing, not only in areas of the forebrain connected with producing movement, but also in the primitive "emotional" cortex and in the amygdala. According to their research, sending the sensory/motor information to an area connected with emotion allowed an expression of empathy.

Even rat brains have the capacity to transfer purely sensory information to an emotionally and ethically important brain region such as the amygdala. In Poland, Ewelina Knapska and Tomasz Werka kept rats in pairs. Within each pair, the "demonstrator" was exposed either to foot shock conditioning or to a neutral novel environment. The visually painful experience of the demonstrators who were shocked affected the behavior of the other, "observer" rats. Those rats that viewed the shocked demonstrators anxiously explored their enclosures more, a significant change in reactive anxiety state that was greater than in the rats that viewed the behavior of non-shocked demonstrators. Knapska and Werka showed that even in rats, sensory information of the sort that in a higher animal would be connected with empathy had been transferred to the amygdala, resulting in a change in emotional behavior.

Many nerve cell circuits can yield outputs that in one state of activity yield a particular positive electrical signal that we could name "S," but in a different state of electrical activity yield the opposite, "Not S." Such circuits act as switches. In the neural circuitry between the amygdala and the prefrontal cortex, I am proposing an "emotional switch" that, for our purposes, exerts a judgment of "good" or "bad." In "one position of the switch," that is, in one state of neuronal activity the intended action will have a positive valence, a pleasant result. However, the switch could be flipped to its other position, if the result of the intended action is understood as having an unpleasant or even harmful result. As a result of this evaluation, an altruistic, prosocial act will be precipitated.

And remember, even though I have cited visual images as factors in ethical decisions, because vision is the paradigm sensory system in humans, none of the steps described are limited to one sensory modality. These sensory modalities, like the auditory, kinesthetic, tactile, and olfactory systems, could follow the same principles.

Genes potentially important. Now, what controls the switch that will determine what kind of message gets sent to neurons in Step 5 of ABT? Recent neuroscience studies already have started to get a handle on genetic mechanisms that can strengthen the tendency of an animal or human to act well toward another individual if the emotional switch says that an action is beneficial to the other. Gene products (each gene's RNA and protein) that are already proven important for controlling social behaviors of people and higher animals toward one another are considered to be the likely causes. The genes coding for the peptide oxytocin (OT) and its specialized receptor (OTR) have received a great deal of scientific attention. I theorize that high OT activity working through OTR in the amygdala and prefrontal cortex would enforce a switch position that yields prosocial behaviors. Other gene products are also involved. For example, vasopressin (VP), a small molecule composed of only nine amino acids, could be important in this regard. Consider also, corticotropin-releasing hormone (CRH), the stress-related neuropeptide with the greatest importance in causing fear and anxiety. It could be involved. Thus, even now, during this initial phase of discovery, we have plenty of molecular candidates to help us do the job of making an ethical decision. The genes, as well as the neural circuit mechanisms already mentioned, are in place to make the Altruistic Brain work.

So Step 4 of the theory, following the several mechanisms for merging of images, proposes the passage of sensory information relevant for a moral decision from the cool, calculated sensory-motor parts of the brain—the "Apollonian nervous system," named after the cerebral Greek god of reason—to parts of the brain connected with roiling emotions, the "Dionysian nervous system" named after the Greek god devoted to sensate desires.

NEURAL BASIS OF STEP 5: THE DECISION AND THE ACT

In Step 5, we complete the process, a classic Yes/No decision that the central nervous system has to make all the time. Carrying out the behavior uses ordinary motor control neurophysiology of the sort that has been studied for almost a century. This is the simplest step of the theory because the emotional valence of the considered act has already been realized. If, in Step 4, the intended action leads to a positive result, then the action will be carried out. If an intended action leads to perceived harm of the imaged self achieved in Step 3, then the action will not be carried out.

Where in the brain does this final step take place? Modern neuroscience's best guess right now would be in a hitherto obscure part of the cerebral cortex called the "insula." Insula neurons respond to pleasant states (leading to the performance of the intended response) or to the impression of moral disgust (leading to abstention from the intended response). The output of the insula connects to motor control systems in the forebrain that allow the insula to "weigh in" on the performance of the motor act that is being considered. If there are good consequences, then it's Go! If, however, there are bad consequences for the act's intended recipient, then it's No Go.

FROM THE DECISION TO SUPPORTING THE ACTUAL, ALTRUISTIC BEHAVIOR

When the decision to perform an altruistic act has been completed, like that of Steven Siller, what neurobiological forces ensure that the act will actually be carried out? Does the brain proceed with the motor act based on "goodness for its own sake," or are there strong biological forces that have evolved to encourage prosocial behavior? The answer is the latter, and those forces are grounded in our instincts toward sex and parental care, that is, in the biology of reproduction. A tremendous amount of primary neuroscience research tells us how this works and we'll examine those studies in Chapter 4.

FURTHER READING

S. Bandyopadhyay, Bernd Sutor, and John J. Hablitz. 2006. "Endogenous Acetylcholine Enhances Synchronized Interneuron Activity in Rat Neocortex." *Journal of Neurophysiology* 95, 1908–1916.

L. Carr, M. Iacoboni, M. C. Dubeau, J. C. Mazziotta, and G. L. Lenzi. "Neural Mechanisms of Empathy in Humans: A Relay from Neural Systems for Imitation to Limbic Areas." *PNAS* 100 (2003), 5497–502.

Katherine Cullen. 2013."Vestibular and Oculomotor Physiology." In Donald Pfaff, ed., *Neuroscience in the 21st Century*, pp. 839–882. Heidelberg and New York: Springer Science+Business Media.

Anthony Damasio. 1999. *The Feeling of What Happens*. San Diego: Harcourt.

Anthony Damasio. 2010. *Self Comes to Mind*. New York: Pantheon.

Frans B. M. de Waal, Marietta Dindo, Cassiopeia A. Freeman, and Marisa J. Hall. 2005. "The Monkey in the Mirror: Hardly a Stranger." *PNAS* 102, 11140–11147.

R. Desimone, T. D. Albright, C. C. Gross, and C. Bruce 1984. "Stimulus Selective Properties of Inferior Temporal Neurons in the Macaque. *Journal of Neuroscience* 4, 2051–2062.

L. Fogassi, Pier Francesco Ferrari, Benno Gesierich, Stefano Rozzi, Fabian Chersi, and Giacomo Rizzolatti. 2005."Parietal Lobe: From Action Organization to Intention Understanding." *Science* 308, 662–664.

V. Gallese, L. Fadiga, L., L. Fogassi, and G. Rizzolatti. 1996. "Action Recognition in the Premotor Cortex." *Brain* 119, 593–609.

C. Gross, C. E. Rocha-Miranda, and D. B. Bender 1972. "Visual Properties of Neurons in Inferotemporal Cortex of the Macaque." *Journal of Neurophysiology* 35, 96–111.

Nancy Kanwisher, Josh McDermott, and Marvin M. Chun. 1997. "The Fusiform Face Area: A Module in Human Extrastriate Cortex Specialized for Face Perception." *Journal of Neuroscience* 17, 4302–4311.

E. Knapska, E. Nikolaev, P. Boguszewski, G. Walasek, J. Blaszczyk, L. Kaczmarek, and T. Werka. 2006. "Between-Subject Transfer of Emotional Information Evokes Specific Pattern of Amygdala Activation." *PNAS* 103, 3858–3862.

Michael V. Lombardo, Bhismadev Chakrabarti, Edward T. Bullmore, Susan A. Sadek, Greg Pasco, Sally J. Wheelwright, John Suckling, MRC AIMS Consortium, and Simon Baron-Cohen. 2010. "Atypical Neural Self-representation in Autism." *Brain* 133, 611–624.

J. McKinstry, Gerald M. Edelman, and Jeffrey L. Krichmar. 2006. "A Cerebellar Model for Predictive Motor Control Tested in a Brain-based Device." *PNAS* 103, 3387–3392.

S. Ohayon, W. Freiwald, and D. Tsao. 2012. "What Makes a Cell Face Selective? The Importance of Contrast." *Neuron* 74, 567–581.

Donald Pfaff. 2007. *The Neuroscience of Fair Play*. New York: Dana Press.

J. Poulet and B. Hedwig. 2006. "The Cellular Basis of a Corollary Discharge." *Science* 311, 518–522.

Rodrigo Quian Quiroga, Lawrence H. Snyder, Aaron P. Batista, He Cui, and Richard A. Andersen. 2006. "Movement Intention Is Better Predicted than Attention in the Posterior Parietal Cortex." *Journal of Neuroscience* 26, 3615–3620.

Justin H.G. Williams, Gordon D. Waiter, Anne Gilchrist, David I. Perrett, Alison D. Murray, and Andrew Whiten. 2006. "Neural Mechanisms of Imitation and 'Mirror Neuron' Functioning in Autistic Spectrum Disorder." *Neuropsychologia* 44, 610–621.

[4]

NEURAL AND HORMONAL
MECHANISMS THAT PROMOTE
PROSOCIAL BEHAVIORS ONCE
THE ETHICAL DECISION
IS MADE

What specific factors provided the mechanistic routes for the evolution of altruistic instincts described in Chapter 1? As any evolutionary biologist will tell you, no complex behavior emerges fully formed and goes from "0 to 60" in a single spurt. Instead, friendly behaviors that evolved to support reproduction provided the substrate that enabled altruistic behaviors reaching beyond the immediate family ultimately to take off. That is, as humans engaged in sex and parenthood—with repeated, intense opportunities for intimacy and caring—they literally practiced, internalized, and then generalized beyond their immediate social sphere the kindness that these behaviors entailed. Sex and parenthood were thus the laboratories where our species learned how to give spontaneously, if for no other reason than that giving was necessary to sustain relationships among partners and children, as well as to sustain the life of helpless infants. In this chapter, I want to explain how sex and parenthood operated, over eons, to imprint an instinct for spontaneous kindness—a.k.a. altruism—on the human brain, so that now it is so much a part of our collective personality that we have ceased to recognize its origin in primitive, but ultimately crucial survival mechanisms.

Yet even though it is part of our species' evolutionary inheritance, I will also argue that kindness is something that we learn, as individuals, as we begin to experience sexual intimacy and parenthood. Kindness is, as it were, reimprinted on our brains as we *choose* it for the pleasurable associations that it entails. Sex and parenthood are thus still at work in our lives in secondary capacities, reinforcing traits that we are already inclined to express.

In Chapter 3, we examined the array of scientific studies that underlie Altruistic Brain Theory (ABT). That chapter showed how without doing anything out of the ordinary—either in terms of the brain's capacity or in terms of how science understands that capacity—the brain can implement the steps leading to altruistic behavior. That is, as a practical matter, well-accepted neuroscience leads to the conclusion that we are "wired" to behave altruistically. Neuroscience understands the *elements* of how we can be altruistic; when these elements are concatenated, as in ABT, our capacity for ethical behavior is not a mystery.

But there is still another question that we need to address. The question involves the nature of choice, and why, once we have processed the information in Steps 1 through 4, we are more likely to act, in Step 5, in a way that benefits another person.

What biological factors in the brain fuel the behaviors that result from the Altruistic Brain's decision? ABT states that once the brain processes the sequence of steps entailed by its "golden rule" wiring, and the potential result of an action is evaluated, an ethical switch flips toward "Yes" or "No." If Yes: a prosocial act is undertaken. If No: an antisocial act is avoided. In either case, the issue is: what is the determinant? Why does someone act or refrain from acting, and why would the action (or failure to act) more likely be toward the decent end of the spectrum as opposed to the nasty? It is important to understand the neurohormonal forces acting in the brain in such a way as to actually produce friendly behaviors (and block unfriendly ones) once the ethical decision has been made. Not only do such prosocial behaviors produce the desired consequences for society and civilized life, but they also promote health because they support friendships. Many medical and epidemiological studies have shown that having friends, on average, prolongs life and increases its quality, as well as improving our psychological well-being. So now we will explore hormonal and neural factors that encourage and support prosocial behaviors when the Altruistic Brain has made the decision to perform a beneficent act.

Consider, for example, an application to a real-life example of the brain mechanisms described in Chapters 1–3. Once Steven Siller's brain went through the first four steps toward an altruistic brain, what natural forces in his body made it easier for him to follow through? That is, what neural mechanisms and biochemicals fostered his turning his altruistic inclination into an actual deed? Backing up a bit, what fundamental qualities in ourselves have evolved over time that make the brain respond, in a positive way, to impulses issuing from the ethical switch? In the view of science, this response—this decision to be altruistic—is rooted in a person's yearning to be together with another human being, that is, to engage in the type of reciprocal acts that contribute to human happiness.

Much of our happiness (or pain) depends on the quality of our social relationships. In fact, there are great advantages to living socially, highlighted, for example, in cooperation to find food and the mutual effort to detect and reduce danger. These advantages drove the evolution of sociality. This chapter argues that the evolution of mechanisms in the brain favoring sociality and, hence, reciprocity, allow the ethical switch to literally turn us on to acting in an ethical, altruistic way. It also argues that acting altruistically produces a profound pleasure on the continuum with that derived from sexuality. Connection with other people is necessary for our sense of well-being. Reciprocity, in the form of reciprocal kindness, is a source of pleasure that we need and even seek. So the basic question, then, is *why* reciprocal kindness makes us happy, and why from an evolutionary perspective nature designed us this way.

While I will provide the scientific answer to this question, we can probably all agree that we feel better in the company of people whom we know to be supportive, and we know that they will more likely be supportive if we support them as well. Community is as old as humanity, as we like the feeling of connection and safety that it provides. Nature designed us to like each other because we are more likely to survive communally.

When we take care of others, displaying our altruistic brains in action, we are using neural circuits and hormonal stimuli that build on those that our evolutionary forerunners established for purposes of mating and taking care of the young. In acting altruistically, we extend our purview far beyond sex partners and our own children to include people to whom we are not even related. In evolutionary terms, we have "learned" from sex and parenting behaviors, thus creating a feedback loop that reinforces our instincts toward ethical behaviors. Put another way, because stimuli from the opposite sex cause us to activate hormonal and neural mechanisms that can issue in erotic acts, and because other stimuli trigger parental instincts, when we act altruistically we extend our actions to encompass many more people as objects of emotionally positive, friendly acts. As you will see, our brains build on and add to these *specific* hormonal and neural mechanisms to achieve a much broader repertoire of civilized, social behaviors. We are wired and hormonally prepared to desire connection; it makes us feel good; and from connection comes reciprocity, the best way to ensure connection in the future. Acting well toward others and their acting well toward us are self-reinforcing, a "virtuous circle." They are self-reinforcing because we like the feeling of treating others well and their treating us well. But where does this social drive come from? How did it originate?

SEX AND PARENTHOOD

We often take sex and parenthood for granted. But we shouldn't, especially insofar as they implicate behavioral patterns not readily identified with them. Sex and parenthood provide the building blocks—hormones, such as estrogens, and neurochemicals such as oxytocin (OT)—for the normal, friendly social behaviors that we desire. Sex and parenthood provide the mechanisms that are needed for a wider variety of social behaviors that then become the subjects of reciprocal transactions. They act as a type of fuel, providing the power—the capacity—for attaining the positive disposition necessary for ethical reciprocity. The brain mechanisms for sex and parenthood empower ABT, and help turn the decision of Step 5 into actual human behavior.

Can it be proven, with the certitude of linear geometry, exactly how social behaviors evolved from sex and parenthood? No. But there is no alternative to this evolutionary path. It was impossible for civilized social behaviors to have sprung up from nothing. Instead, during evolution, sexual rewards followed by the rewards of parenthood formed a trajectory of rewarding social behaviors that culminated in the pleasures of society that we enjoy today as normal human beings. I see the development of reciprocal, even altruistic behaviors as occurring in sequence, based on the progression from sex to motherhood, which along the way impart lessons to the participants concerning the emotional benefits of strong connection.

First, let's look briefly at parenthood and paternal behavior as compared to (one gendered version) maternal behavior. Scientists know that in many species the father plays essential roles in caring for the young. Among some species of birds, for example, the father will forage and bring back food to the nest while the mother sits on the egg(s) and keeps them warm; and then roles are reversed—the father sits on the eggs to keep them warm, and so forth. The mother and father cooperate. And among some species of rodents, paternal care is essential, essentially forcing cooperation between mother and father. Most important to us, of course, is that humans, also, are a "biparental species." We all know of examples of couples in which the father is more nurturing than the mother. Paternal behavior is a big deal. However, with respect to hormonal and brain mechanisms analyzed in laboratory animals, we know much more detail about what is necessary for the mother's behavior than the father's. I suspect that once the male's native testosterone-fueled aggression is damped (how, we don't know), mechanisms for his caring behavior are much like the mother's, but there is still not enough evidence to know that for certain. Therefore, in most of this chapter, I will concentrate on maternal behaviors as their role also is supported by a vast amount of research.

Looking forward, here is the first step in the sequence concerning the progression from sex to motherhood: mammalian animals almost always behave in a friendly way toward each other during courtship and mating. Second step: such animals take care of a needy object during maternal behavior. Third step: generalizing from straightforward care for one's young, we have the concept of communal parenting or "alloparenting," which extends the pleasure of parenting outward within a community. That is the broad overview—the simplest and most primitive urges toward reciprocal behavior start with sex. So, we'll now look at brain mechanisms, beginning with those that were the simplest to figure out, which do not even require governance of the cerebral cortex, followed by the more complicated brain mechanisms of maternal behaviors. This order of complexity of brain mechanism mirrors the biological order, sex before motherhood and that before broader forms of community.

Sex and motherhood provide the pleasure of community that, in higher species, will broaden to include an incredibly wide range of pleasurable and productive social behaviors. Sex and consequent motherhood train us to love intimacy. As babies receiving our parents' care we get our first training for communality on a broader scale. So we do not wait until being parents ourselves to receive the rewards of prosocial, altruistic behavior; rather, the species' evolutionary history of sex and parental mechanisms provide the wherewithal by which prosocial behaviors develop and take place.

All of these social behaviors contribute to the development of more widespread altruistic proclivities consequent to ABT. In turn, reciprocal altruism will work well to sustain such behaviors. Sexual instincts and parental instincts provide the brain's "toolkit" for building positive, communal behaviors.

Sex, the Earliest Reason for Two Animals to Get Together

Why do two animals ever get together? To reproduce. While fish do not need socially intimate sex to produce fry, for mammals the case is different. "Internal fertilization" by mammals requires that the male and the female get together so that the male can deliver the sperm into the female, thus to reach and penetrate the egg. Proximity and coordinated activity are necessary for successful sex.

The elementary building blocks of hormonal and nervous system devices that will support friendly and even altruistic behaviors start in the simplest fashion: hormone secretions and neuronal wiring that produce sex behavior, followed inevitably by parental behavior. Leading the way as the most primitive array of brain mechanisms to support social behaviors are those mechanisms that produce sexual behaviors. I will describe the relevant nerve cells and hormones in some detail so that you can get a sense of how specifically we are designed to seek intimate, sexual contact, a source of intense pleasure. Of particular note: the structures (nerve cells and hormones) that are relevant to the search for intimacy are remarkably similar in all mammals, so when I talk about laboratory animals the same will apply to humans. This is because the neuroanatomy and chemistry of these animals' cells have largely been "conserved" to the human brain; as nature spent millions of years evolving hormonal chemistry, brain anatomy, and physiology that work, nature did not discard them when brains got more complicated in primates and even humans. Instead, nature adds to their complexity and builds around them, regulating primitive behaviors by accommodating a more sophisticated set of social signals. This is true for the female and also for the male.

Hypothalamic Nerve Cells

Just above the roof of the mouth there is a small brain region called the hypothalamus. The hypothalamus first became famous because it controls the secretions from the pituitary gland that hangs off it, the so-called "master gland" whose secretions regulate other glands in the body, such as the ovaries, the testes, the adrenal glands, and the thyroid gland. But it has also become clear that nerve cells in the hypothalamus most powerfully control an array of instinctive behaviors. Because primitive sexual instincts "set things up" for a wider range of prosocial behaviors, let's examine their brain and hormonal mechanisms in some detail.

Among such instinctive behaviors, let's first consider female sexuality. In four-footed animals, including laboratory mice and rats, the female controls all of reproduction by either adopting a sway-backed posture that allows the male to fertilize, or by refusing to adopt that posture. That decision to reproduce or not depends on a small group of cells in the middle of the hypothalamus. If these nerve cells in the hypothalamus are sending large numbers of electrical signals toward the midbrain, then the female response that permits fertilization is possible. If not, then not (Figure 4.1).

Once those signals get to the midbrain, they change the status of a brain region right in the middle of the midbrain called the midbrain central gray. For an entire array of instinctive behaviors, from anger and rage through sleep and sex, the midbrain central gray is "ground zero." My lab found that nerve cells in one corner of the midbrain central gray, when activated, will tell powerful behavior-activating neurons deep in the lower brainstem, just above the spinal cord, to say "Go" to the spinal cord, thus preparing the female for sex behavior. That is, when the male touches the female in the right places, the female will snap into

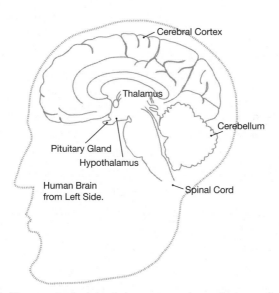

Figure 4.1 Neurons in the hypothalamus not only regulate sexual and social behaviors that are hormone sensitive, but they also regulate the pituitary, the "master gland" that tells other glands (e.g., ovaries, testes, adrenals, thyroid glands) in the body what to do.

the sway-backed posture that allows him to fertilize. If that signal did not originate in the hypothalamus, then it's no go.

On top of this nerve cell "sex circuit," what makes the difference for those hypothalamic neurons, as to whether they will send electrical signals to the midbrain or not? Crucial to that decision are the hormones that tell the hypothalamus what is going on in the rest of the body. In lower animals, especially those that can be preyed upon, running around to find sex is too dangerous to do if the rest of the female's body is not prepared to reproduce. The brain finds out that the female's body is indeed ready to reproduce when the cells of the ovary in the female are ready to ovulate; those ovarian cells will have sent estrogens, into the bloodstream. The estrogens circulate throughout the body, easily get into the brain, and arrive at the hypothalamic neurons. There, the estrogens perform two tasks. They permit those hypothalamic neurons to fire more electrical signals in response to their electrical inputs, and they turn on genes in hypothalamic neurons that further encourage sex behavior. Female sex behavior is even stronger if another hormone arrives in the brain. Progesterone, coming from the ovaries, will multiply the positive effect of estrogens on female sex behavior. So if the estrogens, multiplied by progesterone's effects, have arrived at these hypothalamic neurons, they will respond to their neuronal inputs by firing out electrical signals that activate the rest of the female sex behavior circuit.

What inputs do these hypothalamic cells receive? The most important inputs we have found out so far reflect the overall state of arousal of the brain. For example, the arousing neurotransmitter norepinephrine, a small molecule that will make us hyper-alert to all kinds of stimuli in our environments, will make these hypothalamic cells fire electrical signals. Crystal meth imitates norepinephrine's effects. Likewise, histamine turns on these hypothalamic nerve cells. Think of what an antihistamine does to you: it makes you sleepy. That is because histamine itself wakes us up, and it also makes hypothalamic nerve cells active, to send electrical signals back to the midbrain. In general, chemicals in the nervous system that arouse the brain, activating sex behaviors in these laboratory animals, and those that depress overall brain arousal have opposite effects.

Male sex behaviors in laboratory animals do not depend on the hypothalamus. Instead, a small group of nerve cells just in front of the hypothalamus called the preoptic area (POA) must be working effectively for male sex behavior to be initiated. If the male laboratory animal is to chase after the sexually receptive female and to mount her and fertilize, these cells will have received inputs from the olfactory system signaling the reception of sex hormone–dependent odors from the female. Once activated, these POA neurons send electrical signals down their axons, back to a different part of the midbrain, thus to control brainstem circuits that activate the male's erection and ejaculation.

These POA neurons also depend on hormones. The steroid hormone testosterone, secreted from the testes and circulating throughout the body in the bloodstream, is famous for fueling all kinds of "masculine" behaviors, but now comes the tricky part. In the male's brain, testosterone can be chemically converted into estrogens, and the full range of testosterone's behavioral effects in the brain depends on both hormones. These POA neurons are also turned on by neurotransmitters that signal brain arousal. The neurotransmitter dopamine is famous for activating motor behaviors. This activation is especially impressive when it is directed toward salient stimuli in the environment. Neurons that produce dopamine secrete it into the POA. Of course, a receptive female is certainly a salient stimulus to the male. Thus testosterone and estrogens, operating symphonically in the forebrain, allow dopamine-activated POA neurons to respond to environmental stimuli indicating that a receptive female is near. The male will chase the female, mount, and fertilize. These brain mechanisms comprise a primitive substrate for the male wanting to be near another animal, in this case a female. That is, as mentioned, while the neuronal wiring I introduced in

Chapter 2 and detailed in Chapter 3 encourage altruistic behavior, these primitive sex mechanisms provide the drive, the energy to do so. These animals are strongly motivated to have sex. Whether we are talking about laboratory animals like rats and mice, or animals out in the wild, they will suffer pain to have sex; they will travel to have sex; they will expose themselves to predatory dangers to have sex; they will learn all kinds of arbitrary tasks to have sex. Some psychologists claim that sexual motivation is the most powerful psychological force there is. For purposes of my argument, the main point is that there is an indubitable, irresistible need among animals to literally unite with their kind. The behavior offers a type of pleasure that each individual finds necessary. It comprises the most elementary primitive form of prosocial behavior that provides neural and hormonal mechanisms that fuel togetherness and provide energy for the kind of prosocial act explained by ABT.

Sex Is Just the Beginning

We like sex and, by extension, we are predisposed to like other forms of intimacy and reciprocity. Moreover, as adults we seek other forms of intimacy that play off our enjoyment of sex. Sexual mechanisms have provided the wiring for social behaviors and the neurochemical mechanisms involving estrogens, OT, and the like, to support a wide range of social behaviors. These chemical molecules provide some of the fuel needed to turn ABT into action.

Sex and motherhood train us to love intimacy. The simplest building block in making hormonal supports for social behavior sprang from the requirement for getting male and female together so that sperm could fertilize the egg. The most primitive tie between two laboratory animals or, for that matter, between two human beings is sex. Sex provides the most elementary lesson in how to interact productively. For the female, the inevitable consequence of successful sex will be that she will become a mother.

If sex behaviors are among the simplest social behaviors, then maternal behaviors are among the more complex. Maternal behaviors, in turn, will lead us toward more generally altruistic behaviors toward our kin, neighbors, colleagues, and even strangers.

Mothering

We sometimes say that "maternal love knows no limits." A different set of neurons (from those involved in sex behavior) and a different symphony of hormones flooding into the brain are required for maternal behavior. Because the very first experience of caring behavior will be experienced by the baby at the instigation of the mother, we want to know how this caring behavior works. And when adult humans are following patterns of altruistic behavior according to my theory, you could almost say that the caregiver, the person who is being altruistic, is using some of the same brain and hormonal mechanisms as allow a mother behaving toward a baby. Parenthood offers a "baby step" toward the generally altruistic behaviors that depend on the five steps of ABT.

A female mouse in the laboratory must perform several tasks to take care of her young. First, during late pregnancy, she'll make a nest. Any sort of scraps of paper, leaves, wood, that she can render soft can be woven into the larger part of a hollow sphere, say, about three or four inches in diameter. The nest will help her to keep the young warm and will hide her little family from predators. Then, as she is giving birth to nine or ten babies, some will get out of the nest. The mother has to scurry after them, pick them up gently in her mouth, and get them back into the nest. There, she will lick them extensively, which cleans them and warms them. Huddling over them motionless in a posture that allows them access to her nipples for nursing but does not smother them, she is affording them bodily contact, protection, warmth, and food. For the babies, the extent of this contact with the mother will influence their own social behaviors for the rest of their lives. In laboratory animals and in humans the pleasure of close, nurturant bonds to mom fosters positive social behaviors in later life.

In a special part of the POA, in front of the hypothalamus toward the nose, and well above the bottom of the brain, is a group of neurons that send their signals back toward the midbrain, where they will communicate with a midbrain cell group exquisitely sensitive for controlling a wide range of emotional behaviors. We don't know yet exactly how these maternal behaviors, dependent on preoptic neurons, form a building block for reciprocally altruistic social behaviors. But the import of these preoptic neurons and their connections is at least twofold. First, they permit the chain of behaviors—nest building, retrieving pups, and so forth—that enable the mother to take care of the young. Second, and just as important, they suppress fear and anxiety: fear of the environment and even fear of the strange little objects that we call babies.

As they do so, these neurons will be assisted in their job by a symphony of hormones flooding into the brain from the rest of the body. Supporting maternal behaviors that give pleasure to mother and baby, these hormones "set the stage" for a wider range of mutually supportive social behaviors. Mothers are programmed to be mothers, and hormones are part of the program.

In lab animals and in humans, the mother's level of estrogens will remain high throughout pregnancy and, postpartum, while caring for babies. Progesterone is more complicated. Progesterone stayed at high levels during most of the pregnancy, but it falls to low levels just before the mother gives birth. In fact, it absolutely must fall to low levels for maternal behavior to be expressed. Here, as is so often the case for hormone effects on behavior, the natural pattern is the optimal pattern.

Second, because giving maternal care is much more complicated than sex, it not only needs a wider range of behavioral elements to be successful, but concomitantly a virtual symphony of hormones. Many hormones have to chime in, as well as estrogens and progesterone, to prepare the mother's body for the demands of producing milk. For example, prolactin is a large protein acting as a hormone produced by the pituitary gland and circulating in the mother's bloodstream. Prolactin acts on the breasts and is necessary for normal lactation. Its levels in the blood go up just before birth, and if its secretion is prevented by drug administration, then maternal behavior is delayed. Conversely, administration of prolactin in animals that are deficient maternally will stimulate full maternal behavior (Figure 4.2).

As I just noted, maternal behavior is hormonally more sophisticated than simple sex behavior. For example, cholecystokinin (CCK), a body chemical that stimulates eating behavior, also stimulates maternal behaviors such as building a nest or retrieving pups. CCK, injected into female rats primed with estrogens, quickly stimulates maternal behavior, while blocking CCK actions pharmacologically disrupts maternal behavior. Because CCK can cause the release of prolactin, maybe the routes of CCK action on maternal behavior are indirect.

Maternal behavior falls prey to environmental disruptions that cause fear and anxiety. Laboratory animals are afraid of things that are strange, and to the female mouse, pups are strange. In fact, mothers are required to extend care toward strange little beings that they might at

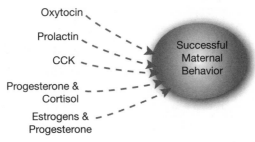

Figure 4.2 Maternal behavior is complicated. More than five hormones are involved in its regulation.

first actually fear. So from this perspective, you can see a role for neurochemicals that would dull the feelings of fear. Chemicals that act like opium—so-called opioid peptides—do just that. They act through opioid receptors in the brain. Block those opioid receptors and you'll find that, starting from the birth of the pups, the mother's behavior is deficient. She does not clean them as she should just after birth, and the other maternal behaviors described previously are delayed. In fact, Cambridge professor Barry Keverne, a pioneer in the study of behavioral biology, found that caregiving and protective behaviors by monkeys also were reduced when opioid receptors were blocked, supporting the basic idea that maternal behaviors lie at the evolutionary basis of many positive, prosocial behaviors. In hospitals, I have witnessed the same phenomenon among women, as when pharmaceuticals that help nursing women relax and reduce anxiety or pain also help them to continue nursing. So neurochemicals that reduce fear and anxiety enhance maternal behaviors and other forms of caregiving.

For maternal behaviors, oxytocin (OT) is the neurochemical that is the star of our show. Cort Pedersen, who both practices clinical psychiatry and does academic research at the University of North Carolina, discovered that when OT is administered to the brain of female rats who had not acted maternally, maternal behavior would suddenly appear. Then Susan Fahrbach, when a student in my lab at Rockefeller University, found that blocking OT receptors—proteins on the surface of neurons, specialized to bind OT in a way that changes neuronal functions—in female rats that had been maternal would significantly reduce their maternal behaviors. They did not retrieve their pups and did not assume a nursing posture. A large number of scientific papers since those by Pedersen and Fahrbach have confirmed that in female mammals that have estrogens on board, OT is a major player among the neurochemicals that foster maternal care.

In addition to the nerve cell pathways from the POA, a large number of hormonal and neurochemical supports for maternal behaviors guarantees that they will be carried out successfully. Estrogens, progesterone, prolactin, CCK, opioids, serotonin, and OT all play their roles. Maternal behaviors are such important behaviors that they are overdetermined: several independent causes overlap in various combinations, safeguarding behaviors and making sure that they occur.

British behavioral biologist Barry Keverne has written extensively on the developmental and evolutionary roots of social behaviors. Indeed, he has addressed the theory that, after sex, the relationship between mother and child is the most basic that any of us ever experience. He queries how secure the infant/mother attachment is in early life, and suggests that it has enormous predictive value: "anxious attachments (between mother and child) may be conceived as a risk factor for subsequent socio-emotional problems." A shaky relationship foreshadows "more difficult, aggressive peer relationships and few good, close friends." Nature, however, has evolved brain mechanisms that foster strong mother/child attachments and ensure that such attachments give us pleasure. Such pleasure becomes paradigmatic. As we grow, our capacity to form bonds grows with us, becoming more complex as new relationships provide more scope for us to derive pleasure from attachment. Notably, even though we are not conscious as babies of giving pleasure to our mothers, we are—even as babies—already involved in a reciprocal relationship where we derive support and provide gratification; our mothers literally love feeding us and watching us grow. Of course, babies already do their part to establish a reciprocal relationship by gazing at their mothers, cooing, smiling, and even imitating their mothers.

An important brain mechanism that allows us to bond with our mothers and later, with our friends, requires the production and synaptic release of brain chemicals that have opium-like effects. These chemicals are called "endogenous opioids" because they are in the brain (as opposed to outside), and calm us down the way opium or heroin would. The mother triggers their release, in Keverne's view, by intense and continuous touching, or "grooming" the baby, thus calming it. We see this extensively in laboratory animals. Even more impressive is that primates benefit from this kind of care (i.e., continuous touching of other animals, especially of infants by mothers) extending long into childhood. Such extended care from our mothers is necessary for the ability to form normal relationships.

EVOLUTIONARY PERSPECTIVE

Now let's view all these scientific details from an evolutionary perspective. The "biological engineering" problems that must be overcome to achieve reproduction by mammals can be understood by comparisons to lower forms such as fish. In evolutionary terms, how do land-based mothers prepare for reproduction, having advanced from fish-like water-borne reproduction (no intimate contact)? A mother uses her large mammalian brain, as Keverne writes, to plan ahead, for example, "increasing her food intake early in pregnancy enabling reserves to be laid down to meet the extra demands of the exponential growth of her offspring later in pregnancy and for the production of milk needed for post-partum lactation."

Once reproduction is accomplished, the next step can be taken to achieve larger degrees of social organization. In Keverne's words, our living in large social groups "has required the emancipation of parenting behavior from the constraints of hormonal state and the evolution of large brains for decision making that was previously restricted and determined by hormonal state." "The starting point for understanding all bonded relationships is in the conserved mechanisms that underpin mother-infant bonding." Keverne's thinking and observations are incredibly important because they account for how we moved from hormone-dominated parental behaviors to learned social behaviors in large communities.

From Life with Mother to Life with Others

On our way toward explaining the biological urges that help to promote the altruistic behavior that follows on from ABT, we started with the most primitive behaviors: sex and motherhood. Both require attachment to others. The "attachment theory" developed by British psychoanalyst John Bowlby builds on this biological requirement, generalizing from the mother/child bond to demonstrate the importance of such early emotional relations to proper personality formation and to fostering nurturant relations between adults. Coming from a psychological perspective, Bowlby reached conclusions similar to those of Keverne, who employs a more purely biological approach.

Because the instinct for attachment provides important support to the Altruistic Brain's operation, and because Bowlby dominates the academic study of attachment, I will describe his views in some detail. Distinguishing his thinking from Freud's, Bowlby focuses on the *initial* development of attachment between two humans—"how a very young child behaves towards his mother, both in her presence and especially in her absence"—and on what such observations tell us about the development of human social proclivities. He charts the development of attachment behavior by the baby toward the mother, starting with the time that the baby's sensory capacities barely detect and distinguish the mother right through when the baby can move toward the mother and signal to her, to the final phase during which the baby "forms a goal-oriented partnership" with the mother and is able to intuit her feelings and motives.

Bowlby cites conditions that work in both directions to foster attachment behavior between mother and baby. These include influences of the baby on the mother: if the baby does not exhibit cranky behaviors that annoy her, and if the baby actively reaches out toward her, all should be well. Equally important are influences of the mother on the baby: her "early acceptance of a nurturant role" leading to significant physical contact, gentle holding, soothing, and encouragement, "the provision of materials and experiences suited to baby's individual capacities," and "the frequency and intensity of expression of positive feelings toward him." Some of these factors easily find their adult equivalents, and could help to support Altruistic Brain operation in the regulation of social behavior. The result, to use Bowlby's phrase, can be the "persistence and stability of patterns" of social behavior that allow Altruistic Brain operations to produce regular, predictable prosocial behavior without being derailed by adverse neurochemical or even social or cultural conditions.

Bowlby and Keverne are thus two sides of the same coin in that both explain how early experiences foster nurturant relationships among adults. All by itself, OT justifies Keverne's proposition, referred to at the beginning of this chapter, that sex and especially maternal behavior set the stage for brain mechanisms that support a wide range of prosocial behaviors. OT is crucial. From the beginning of life, OT helps with attachment behavior in human infants, increases trust between adults, and can even be used therapeutically. Experimental results from large numbers of studies paint the picture that OT fosters many, many positive social behaviors.

One scientist began his study of maternal behavior with little rats that had not yet even been weaned from the mother. He wanted to find out if, as these tiny animals huddled together, they would show a preference for a scent (lemon or orange) associated with the mother. They did show that preference, but the preference was disrupted if the brain was bathed in a chemical that blocked OT receptors (OTRs). In a long series of studies, Larry Young, a molecular neurobiologist, showed not only the role of OT in promoting friendly side-by-side sitting together by experimental animals, but also the importance of OT binding to receptors in the basal forebrain for mediating this action on social behavior. Inga Neumann, a neuroendocrinologist at the University of Regensburg in Germany, showed that OT helped laboratory animals to overcome the effects of a social defeat, thus restoring a normal degree of social exploration and social preference. Conversely, blocking OTRs had the opposite effect. Many skilled behavioral biologists are convinced that among laboratory animals the performance of maternal behaviors has a lot to do with the mother's innate social anxiety. Female rats bred for a high level of anxiety "displayed an intense and protective mothering style" not shown by females bred for a low level of anxiety. OT fosters maternal behavior by reducing this anxiety through its release in a cell group in the hypothalamus specialized for fearful and anxious reactions to the environment. OT binds maternal behaviors and a broader range of social behaviors together, and the reduction of social anxiety may be part of the trick. The very same chemical, OT, is produced by the very same neurons in the human brain, and travels the same paths to its targets, with the predicted results.

Oxytocin and Social Behavior in General

In people, as well, OT affects social behavior from infancy. A large study of infants in Germany showed that the DNA that makes the OTR influences how well the infants are behaviorally attached to their mothers. A particular line-up of DNA nucleotides (elementary units of DNA) maximized what the investigators called "attachment security," infants' apparent confidence in their mothers' enduring care.

OT also enforces caring behavior. Paul Zak and his team at Claremont Graduate University ran economic games in which subjects could earn money, but also were given chances to donate part of their earnings to charity. Among those subjects who did decide to donate, those who received infusions of OT gave an amazing 48% more to charity than those who received infusions of a placebo control. Not only that, but in laboratory economic games, people who declared that they intentionally displayed trust toward other, anonymous players, had higher levels of OT circulating in their blood. A leading team of

Swiss researchers said that "the effect of OT on trust is not due to a general increase in the readiness to bear risks. On the contrary, OT specifically affects an individual's willingness to accept *social* risks" as a result of the individual's trusting behavior. In fact, one particular genetic variation in the DNA that codes for OTR is reliably associated with trusting behavior. In France, Elissar Andari and his colleagues were so impressed by the increase in social interactions caused by inhaled OT that they suggested it as a possible therapeutic agent to combat the social maladies of autism, as I will document shortly. Adult males studied by Jennifer Bartz were asked to assess their mothers' childhood care. After these males received OT treatment delivered intranasally, they reported their mothers as more caring and close. Their memory of social life with their mothers had a warmer tone.

But OT's effects on social behavior have limits. Its effects on social memory—the ability to remember that you have had friendly relations with another before—appeared most obviously in less anxious subjects. Moreover, OT may promote trust and cooperation within a defined social group but also encourage a defensive sort of aggression during behavior toward an out-group. In some economic games played by subjects in the laboratory, the ability of OT to enhance cooperative behaviors depended on the subjects having a high degree of social information. When the subjects became familiar with other players, the predicted effects of OT to encourage cooperation appeared. When they didn't, neither did the effects. So a massive amount of research with humans shows the prosocial effects of OT, albeit such effects have their limits.

Oxytocin in the Amygdala

How, exactly, does OT produce all these effects that promote social behavior? Some evidence points at the amygdala. The amygdala has more subdivisions than you usually read about, and rather than describe them all I will focus on the most important one for our present point. That is the central nucleus of the amygdala, whose outputs are crucial for our sense of fear and anxiety. A team of Swiss physiologists has recently demonstrated how OT's specific inhibitory effects on these central amygdala neurons also block the freezing responses of laboratory rats to stimuli that trigger sudden fear. These fear-provoking stimuli should include social stimuli, and assuming this is true, we would understand how the effects of OT in the amygdala promote social behavior. In human subjects as well, different parts of the amygdala play different roles. Most important for us, a group of German physicians reported that in the anterior amygdala, OT attenuated responses to fearful faces but increased activity in response to happy facial expressions. In fact, patients with damage to the amygdala on both sides of their brain were impaired in their OT-sensitive social responses. All of these results tell us that the amygdala participates importantly in positive, prosocial responses to positive social stimuli.

In addition, genetic evidence points to the importance of OT signaling for human social behavior. The most telling results have come from studies of people in whom the tiniest element of the genetic code for the OTR has been changed by nature. In one set of experiments, just one such change, a single small chemical unit in DNA, significantly affected a person's empathy. A more complicated set of experiments got similar results, but found that the effect of the OTR gene code on an affiliative behavior, namely seeking emotional support, depended on the subjects being quite distressed. In fact, according to a top group of German scientists, the ability of subjects to benefit from social support depended on the exact DNA sequence of the OTR gene.

In the nervous system, actions of OT on behavior depend on some groups of neurons and not others. For example, with respect to effects on ordinary social behavior, these behavioral effects of OT gene differences are likely to depend on OT projections from the hypothalamus to the amygdala. As pointed out by many neuroscientists, these social effects of the OT/OTR system are especially striking during reproduction, but spread to the rest of social life as well. In sum, if tiny changes in the genetic coding for the OTR are so important, then likewise, we can easily understand the important impact of OT itself, the neurochemical that binds to OTR in the brain, on ethical, prosocial behaviors.

Put all of these chemical supports for maternal behaviors together—estrogens, progesterone, prolactin, CCK, opioids, OT—and you reach the conclusion that though maternal behaviors are complex and demanding, they are so important that they cannot be allowed to fail. Another building block for the altruistic behavior dependent on ABT is in place. Remember, I do not think that altruistic behavior just emerged all at once in the mammalian brain. Instead, it was evolution that came up with the neural wiring and the hormone responsiveness that got animals together for purposes of reproduction. As a result, you are part way to altruism itself, and the purely altruistic behavior will now depend on evolving the brain mechanisms summarized in Chapter 2 and documented in Chapter 3.

Alloparenting

In many species, including our own, females do not restrict their care of infants to their own babies. One version of this pattern of behavior is called "alloparenting," whose word roots mean "other/parenting." For example, a grandmother could give a great deal of care to the infant. Or an older sister could do so, thus giving her practice so that when she becomes pregnant she'll be a better mother to her own children.

Sarah Hrdy, at University of California Davis, is a primatologist whose book, *Mothers and Others,* crystallized our thinking about adults who take care of other peoples' babies. Hrdy was stimulated by naturalists from Charles Darwin to Edward O. Wilson, who thought about societies with high levels of cooperative behavior, and she starts by hinting that alloparenting is nothing special: birds do it, mice do it. However, primate behavior raises the bar or, as Hrdy states: "Like other primates, humans find babies irresistible." The baby's large head relative to the rest of the body, large eyes, pudgy cheeks, short limbs, and clumsy movements do the trick. And, of course, primate infants are all born with abilities far short of what they need to survive. So it is good that in the typical human case, our usual social organization arranges for the baby to be born near kin.

A different pattern of behavior in which females take care of other mothers' babies is called "cooperative breeding" or "communal breeding." These refer to social systems in which the females who are taking care of others' infants are doing so specifically at the expense of their own opportunities for reproduction. For example, in societies that are highly structured in a manner that permits only a small percentage of females to reproduce, the "helper females" doing the communal breeding may be relatives of the dominant female whose own attempts at reproduction have not been successful. Remember the "kin selection" idea from Chapter 1? This example of communal breeding would fit the kin selection principle because the helper female, related to the alpha female mother, is arranging for some of her own DNA to be passed on to the next generation. In any case, it seems clear that the capacity of the group for survival will be greater if females otherwise unemployed help to ensure survival of the young within the group.

Thus instinctual behaviors that evolved to ensure reproduction have "spilled over" into other areas of our lives. That is, in this discussion, as we have moved from strictly sexual behaviors to parental behaviors to alloparenting, you can see that we have come part of the way from primitive instincts that serve reproduction toward prosocial behaviors that generally benefit other members of the same group and the species. We can care for strangers in the same way as we care for ourselves.

In a way, accounting for reciprocal ABT-dependent social behaviors in humans can be analogized to building a cathedral. To build such an edifice we must choose suitable ground; know how to cut stone; how to mortar the stones together; how to keep the roof from falling in. These are separate, essential steps in the building process. By analogy, mechanisms involved in sex and parental behaviors provide essential elements to "building" the complex construction that comprises human prosocial behavior.

Social Drive

As I have argued, social motivations and instincts originate in sexual and maternal behaviors. These primitive behaviors supplied some of the building blocks—hormonal and neuronal stepping stones—toward more subtle and complex human relationships. That is, we understand a process in which humans generalize from behavior toward a sex partner, to babies, to other people's babies, to neighbors at large. These elementary social motivations provide the underlying dispositions that permit ABT mechanisms to guide prosocial behavior.

But if we know something about where prosocial behaviors came from, what makes them rewarding for us right now? Offering a partial answer to this question, neuroscientists in Oregon found that using functional magnetic resonance imaging (fMRI), the idea of charitable giving lights up the "reward center" in the human forebrain. The reward signal in this nerve cell group just in front of the hypothalamus looked, to the neuroscientists doing these studies, indistinguishable from the way other brain reward signals, such as that involving food to a hungry person, would look. This fact in itself gives some insight as to exactly *why* people do good *when* they do good, that is, these scientists could see the potential neuronal basis for charitable, altruistic behavior being intrinsically rewarding.

It seems impossible to overestimate the strength of physiological support for social connections among people. Consider that in addition to all of the bonding between the pregnant mother and her unborn child, the baby's heart rate may actually synchronize with his mother's. In fact, increased maternal stress and anxiety will correlate with increased heart rate in her baby. Close, loving relationships actually foster our physical well-being by lessening stress, giving our autonomic nervous systems—our viscera—a rest, and being intrinsically rewarding. And they are rewarding. According to top neurochemists in the field, one of the jobs of OT is to strengthen the effects of dopamine, a well-known mediator of psychological reward. Positive social experiences "light up" a reward center in the basal forebrain. The anthropologist Helen Fisher, from Rutgers University, put subjects in the fMRI scanner and instructed them to visualize the person who has been the object of their intense love. As a control condition, to provide a non-loving comparison, they imagined neutral figures. Love imagery lit up the reward systems of their primitive basal forebrains, the same neural regions as monetary reward. And, as Barry Keverne has surmised, if positive, prosocial relations were restricted to mother and child among us primate species, we would not survive.

Elena Choleris and I determined how this desire for social approach works in female laboratory animals. The story links four specific genes with social behavior and shows how they work together. One estrogen receptor gene, alpha, produces the estrogen receptor that turns on the gene for the OTR. The other estrogen receptor gene, beta, turns on the gene for OT itself. When both OT and its receptor, OTR, are in the brain in quantity, they can work together to promote prosocial behaviors (Figure 4.3).

So reasoning from the rationale of Chapter 2, when we pursue our desire for social affinities we lose the distinction between ourselves and others. We have gained the opportunity to pursue these social affinities by generalizing from our sex partners and our offspring to others with whom we will be friendly and behave well. The links between reproductive instincts and altruistic behavior are strong in two respects. First, when evolution generated the brain wiring and

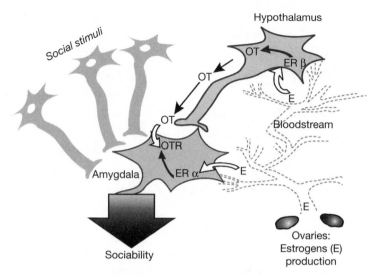

Figure 4.3 In females, four genes in the brain cooperate to foster sociability as it is enhanced by estrogenic (E) hormones. Estrogen, circulating in the blood, is bound by the product of the estrogen receptor beta gene (ER-beta) in certain hypothalamic neurons and is also bound by a product of the estrogen receptor alpha gene (ER-alpha) in amygdala neurons. As a result, in those hypothalamic neurons, oxytocin (OT) is produced, and it travels down the axon to be released and to bind to the oxytocin receptor (OTR) in amygdala neurons. The OTR had been produced there under the influence of ER-alpha.

hormonal responsiveness for sex and maternal behaviors it provided the seedbed for generating generalized altruistic behaviors. Second, the very act of doing courtship, mating, and parental behaviors provides a form of practice for altruistic behavior in general.

WRAP UP, WITH A WARNING

This chapter, based on the biochemistry of hormones as well as on neurochemicals like OT, has shown how decisions to favor prosocial acts, reached via Altruistic Brain mechanisms, are reinforced by primitive, powerful circuitry in the brain. Hormones and nerve cells that regulate the behaviors that are essentially social and that can be among the friendliest behaviors—sex and parenting—provide the evolutionary and mechanistic background for prosociality.

All these scientific findings tell us how various hormones and chemicals facilitate a wonderfully wide range of human behaviors that we all would call "friendly." In fact, once the Altruistic Brain mechanisms make the decision to initiate an altruistic act, hormones and neurons discussed in this chapter propel us to carry out that act, that is, to do the right thing.

Yet notwithstanding these physical predispositions toward prosocial behavior, there are too many circumstances in which people behave in an *antisocial* manner: violent behavior, psychopathology, corruption, and so forth. As you will see in Chapter 6, science knows some of the reasons for such behaviors. This knowledge can, of course, allow us to think about how to address antisocial behaviors by applying Altruistic Brain principles.

FURTHER READING

Jorge A. Barraza, Michael E. McCullough, Sheila Ahmadi, and Paul J. Zack. 2011. "Oxytocin Infusion Increases Charitable Donations Regardless of Monetary Resources." *Hormones and Behavior* 60, 148–151.

J. Bowlby. 1969. *Attachment.* New York: Basic Books. (reprinted 2000).

Elena Choleris, Donald W. Pfaff, and Martin Kavaliers, eds. 2012. *Oxytocin, Vasopressin and Related Peptides in the Regulation of Behavior.* Cambridge, UK: Cambridge University Press.

J. P. Curley and E. B. Keverne. 2005. "Genes, Brains and Mammalian Social Bonds." *Trends in Ecology and Evolution* 20, 561–567.

H. Fisher, L. l. Brown, Aron A. Strong, and D. Mashek. 2010. "Reward, Addiction and Emotion Regulation Systems Associated with Rejection in Love." *Journal of Neurophysiology* 104, 51–60.

Sara Hrdy. 2009. *Mothers and Others.* Cambridge, MA: Harvard University Press.

H. Sophie Knobloch, Alexandre Charlet, Lena C. Hoffmann, Marina Eliava, Sergey Khrulev, Ali H. Cetin, Pavel Osten, Martin K. Schwarz, Peter H. Seeburg, Ron Stoop, and Valery Grinevich. 2012. "Evoked Axonal Oxytocin Release in the Central Amygdala Attenuates Fear Response." *Neuron* 73, 553–556.

I. Neumann and E. H. van den Burg. "Oxytocin and Vasopressin Release and Their Receptor-mediated Intracellular Pathways that Determine Their Behavioral Effects." In E. Choleris, Donald W. Pfaff, and Martin Kavaliers, eds., *Oxytocin, Vasopressin and Related Peptides in the Regulation of Behavior*, pp. 27–43 Cambridge, UK: Cambridge University Press.,

Donald Pfaff. 2005. *Brain Arousal and Information Theory*. Cambridge, MA: Harvard University Press.

Donald Pfaff. 2010. *Man and Woman: An Inside Story*. New York: Oxford University Press.

[5]

NEW NEUROSCIENCE
RESEARCH

The Theory's Link to an Ethical Universal

This chapter links Altruistic Brain Theory (ABT) to the latest neuroscience research on ethical decision making. That research, in turn, sheds light on the biological origins of classical morality. I will argue that there is a discernible path to the laboratory from Buddha, the Bible, and the great 19th century philosophers. My point, therefore, will be that ABT is an explicit, scientific approach to ideas that have persisted in culture for a very long time. What is new is the science.

So let's start with the research on ethical decision making to which ABT is linked. Chapter 4 showed how, for Altruistic Brain Step 4 to work, brain representations of intended motor acts (from ABT Step 1) had to converge with the merged sensory images of self and other (from ABT Step 3). This convergence occurs in neurons in the prefrontal cortex (refer to Figure 2-1). Insofar as it concerns this area of the brain, the theory dovetails with some of the most innovative research in modern neuroscience, which uses new technology to examine the cortex in context with ancient philosophical ideas.

IN THE BRAIN SCANNER

Harvard psychologist Joshua Greene's studies of the human prefrontal cortex pioneered the use of brain scanning to contrast neuronal activity corresponding to "moral sentiments" with motivations that reflect the Utilitarian philosophies of John Stuart Mill, Jeremy Bentham, and others. A Utilitarian approach aims for the greater good for the greatest number, or as in Greene's case, the lesser evil, and tries to save the greater number of would-be victims—*no matter the means*. On the other hand, "moral sentiments" or emotional responses may cause revulsion at the thought of being the direct cause of another person's death. Moreover, not only does Greene invent ingenious laboratory experiments that probe the basis of people's moral decisions, but he also scans their brains during the decision-making process. In this way, he and his fellow researchers analyzed which brain mechanisms support the ethical judgments that people actually make.

As Greene and I have both, in our respective fields, been investigating similar questions, I talked with him during one recent summer. So let's take a look at the clues that his research adds to our understanding of the essential goodness of human nature.

The field of behavioral neuroscience has just entered an era when questions that used to be dealt with only by philosophers can now be brought into the domain of neuroanatomy and behavioral experimentation. Greene is perhaps the brightest and best known researcher to use modern brain-scanning techniques to probe philosophic problems. In his mid-30s, he teaches courses such as "Free Will, Responsibility, and Law" and "Social Neuroscience." His devotion to his field of moral psychology is apparent; he speaks of his field's recent findings with an intensity and level of vitality rarely matched in academic life.

In his lab, Greene takes classic problems in moral philosophy, asks clever questions about that problem, and then turns it into a neuroanatomical investigation. Here is such a problem, first stated by the British philosopher Philippa Foote, summarized briefly by Greene:

"A runaway trolley is hurtling down the tracks toward five people who will be killed if it proceeds on its present course. You can save these five people by diverting the trolley onto a different set of tracks, one that has only one person on it, but if you do this that person will be killed. Is it morally permissible to turn the trolley and thus prevent five deaths at the cost of one?" Philippa Foote's trolley is not presented here as "a perfect moral dilemma," but instead as an intellectual vehicle that helps laboratory scientists achieve basic insights into how ABT operates.

Greene contrasts the foregoing problem to an alternative that asks people to imagine the same setup but, instead of flipping a switch to turn the train, you must personally push a large person in front of the train to stop it from hitting the five people. People often have different reactions to these scenarios, even though the outcomes are the same: five dead or one dead. For most people, it is easier to be Utilitarian in Foote's trolley scenario, where only a switch needs to be thrown and subjects can act at a distance from the inevitable murder. But when it gets "up-close and personal," and test subjects envision physically laying their hands on someone and pushing him into harm's way, most people get queasy and become divided over which is the morally correct choice. Obviously, this is not a rational response. In both scenarios, one person is being sacrificed for the greater good. So what is going on in the second scenario? Emotions are taking over and causing responses that are likely rooted in our evolutionary past.

Greene argues that "humans have inherited many of our social instincts from our primate ancestors," and that these instincts have important emotional components that include severe limitations on our ability to harm one another. These emotional components are faster and more robust than our rational, higher order intellectual processes, making it truly difficult to hurt someone. There are exceptions, of course (and we'll get to those), but when people argue that war and violence are part of our fundamental nature, they may need to take a closer look at the human brain.

While employing a type of brain scanner called a functional magnetic resonance imaging (fMRI) machine, Greene asks human subjects to consider various moral dilemmas and make decisions about what they would do. He varies the emotional intensity of each dilemma (i.e., touching versus acting at a distance) while also changing the weights of the decision (such as saving 10 or 12 people rather than 5) to better probe the factors leading a person to act in a certain way. While subjects are pondering these dilemmas and arriving at decisions, he records relative activity in different regions of their brains.

It turns out that when people are faced with dilemmas where it is easy to choose in a way that would make a Utilitarian proud—that is, they can save the greater number of people using relatively impersonal means, such as throwing a switch—there is greater activation in a brain region known to be involved with abstract thinking and other high-order thought processes called the dorsolateral prefrontal cortex (DLPFC). Specifically, Greene and his colleagues have found that the DLPFC is associated with rational judgments made in the context of competing emotional responses—such as the need to save five people and the revulsion at killing one. This is generally consistent with previous research that depicts the DLPFC as a region responsible for applying "executive" behavioral rules in the face of powerful but unaligned stimuli. (Despite the danger of sounding like we are corporatizing areas of the brain, sometimes neuroscientists borrow terms from business to clarify functions in the brain; regions that serve "executive" functions weigh all the information coming at them from their "inferiors," such as more sensory-focused neurons, and arrive at one course of action over another.)

In a nearby but distinct brain region, the medial (or middle) prefrontal cortex, there is greater activity when the moral judgments are particularly emotional and physically immediate. As an example of such a judgment, let's take a real-life scenario experienced in Nazi Germany. Imagine you are hiding in a confined space with a group of 30 friends and family. You are all frozen-silent, as any sound could lead directly to your deaths. Your infant starts to fuss. You know that the only way to keep her silent for long enough is to smother her. What do you do? Such decisions involve activity of neurons in the medial prefrontal cortex.

Greene and colleagues have also found that the underside, or ventral, area of the medial prefrontal cortex (VMPFC) is involved with tracking the overall value of various outcomes consequent to different actions in response to an ethical choice. Linking this important function of value estimation to ABT, neurons in the VMPFC (according to Josh Greene's new data) can calculate the beneficence (or potential evil) of the intended action (from ABT Step 1) and, according to the result of that calculation, pass on the ABT decision to neurons involved in activating behavior (i.e., neurons that will carry out Step 5 of ABT as introduced in Chapter 2 and detailed in Chapter 3).

As Greene explained to me, "our research is not just showing that the VMPFC is 'involved' in moral judgment in some vague way. Rather, we show that parts of the VMPFC specifically track the statistical interaction between outcome magnitude (i.e., how many lives?) and outcome probability (i.e., what are the odds of saving them?) in the context of moral judgment." He went on to point out how the finding is parallel to previous studies that have used food and monetary rewards rather than "number of lives saved." "This region seems to keep track of expected value more generally," he says. Interestingly, over the course of evolution, both the DLPFC and the VMPFC have grown to impressive sizes in humans and other highly intelligent and social species, such as apes. It could be that the original ability to evaluate prospective food sources was co-opted to also evaluate other important resources, including behaviors that increase social welfare. The importance of these additional skills may have, through the processes of natural selection, resulted in the growth of these areas. This explanation is still speculative, but regardless, the primacy of evolutionarily ancient emotions in making moral "do-no-harm" decisions provides compelling support for the idea that we are born programmed for goodwill.

GOOD AND FAST, FAST AND GOOD

Josh Greene's newest studies have gone further into new sets of experiments, beyond the problems we've addressed so far. Working with his Harvard colleagues David Rand and Martin Nowak, he has used economic games in the lab to explore the manner in which individuals help others even at a cost to themselves. In their so-called "Public Goods Game," 212 subjects recruited from around the world were asked to contribute to a common endowment. All money thus contributed was doubled and then split among the game players. But here is the key result: subjects who made their decisions very fast about how much to contribute were substantially more generous than subjects who made their decisions slowly. Moreover, in Greene's words, "forcing subjects to decide quickly increases contributions, whereas instructing them to reflect and forcing them to decide slowly decreases contributions." In a related experiment, arranging the experimental design such that subjects could "trust their intuition" when contributing to an endowment increased the sizes of their contributions.

In the authors' words, "our first instinct is to cooperate." The automatic, rapid intuitive nature of generous, trusting behavior revealed by Greene, Rand, and Nowak's study underlines and supports ABT that this behavior is built into our brains.

SO YOUNG YET SO GOOD

Other studies of the science underlying altruism examine its development during a human lifetime. Indeed, ABT says that altruism develops early, easily, and naturally, and that it uses an extremely efficient set of neural mechanisms as introduced in Chapter 2 and detailed in Chapter 3. But how deep inside the human psyche does this instinct toward prosocial behavior live? Is it characteristic of particularly sensitive individuals—for example, grade-school teachers—who have spent years honing their responses? No! Even babies have been shown to prefer goodness, as demonstrated in experiments involving games. Games, by definition, are exercises in norms for proper, rule-following behavior. Every game provides a context in which certain rules govern behavior. As predicted by ABT, young children easily adopt these norms because they already come equipped with the requisite brain circuitry.

Michael Tomasello, co-director of the Max Planck Institute of Evolutionary Anthropology in Leipzig, Germany, along with Hannes Rakoczy and their colleagues, taught toddlers novel games and then watched the children's reactions when a puppet played the game incorrectly. For example, in one experiment, there was a play area marked by a blanket on the floor where a child and an experimenter used a sponge in its usual way, pretending to clean up spills and wash dishes. The adult then brought the child and the sponge to another play area, a table, where a new game, dubbed "baffing," was demonstrated using the sponge. Here, the sponge was thrown like dice; the color that landed face side up determined the next step of the game. If it was green, the player got to put a bead onto a string; if it was yellow, the player would not get a bead and the sponge was thrown again.

After the young child got the hang of the game, the experimenter would move away and bury her nose in a book. Then a puppet would come in and use the sponge incorrectly, wiping things up at the baffing table. Here's the point: in some of the experiments as many as two-thirds of the three-year-olds would spontaneously protest, saying things like "No, you are not allowed to clean up here" or "I'll show you how to do it; look it goes like this." In the control condition, the puppet performed the same action—wiping with the sponge—but now the puppet did it in the correct context, on the blanket. Almost none of the children objected in this case.

Such experiments demonstrate that even toddlers quickly understand and follow new social norms—and also apparently assign them significant weight. The ease with which they do so leads directly to the ABT brain mechanisms, and indeed there is a growing number of studies proving that children younger than two years of age already exhibit helping behavior, have a sense of fairness, and can recognize the perspectives and goals of others.

One of the most recent findings along this line was by experimental psychologists Karen Wynn, Paul Bloom, and their colleagues in a powerfully well-equipped child study center at Yale. The researchers created simple characters by giving geometric shapes "googly" eyes. There was a red circle named Climber that would, while an infant watched, get halfway up a hill and celebrate by doing a little dance. Climber would then try to get the rest of the way up, but fail. Twice. Then Helper would come along to give Climber a push up the rest of the hill. Alternatively, Hinderer would show up and shove Climber further down the hill. After watching many such scenes, babies were given a chance to show a preference for either Helper or Hinderer. The babies liked Helper more, by far. Control experiments were done with similar scenes, except the social cues were removed; eyeless shapes simply moved up or down the hill. In these cases, no significant preferences were displayed, suggesting that the children were already thinking in terms of kindness toward shapes that they associated with people.

Indeed, over a series of studies with progressively younger children, researchers have so far been unable to find an age that did *not* show a preference for the prosocial helping shape in comparison to the antisocial one. Even infants as young as three months old disliked the shape that thwarted Climber's efforts. (For the youngest babies, preference was measured by comparing how long the infant looked at each character; duration of eye gaze is a standard measure that has been shown to correlate with verbalized preference at older ages.) Though this may seem like an obvious finding—"babies prefer kindness!"—it is important to note that their judgments are based on actions involving a third party (Climber) rather than themselves. Presumably, the infants were able to take Climber's perspective and have some sense of its intentions and desires. These findings could be interpreted as early displays of empathy and even goal sharing, suggesting these skills do not require special training. Altruism likely is built in, as ABT proposes.

Several additional studies by psychologists have reported that at least under some conditions, children show greater signs of happiness as they are giving their treats to others compared to when receiving the treats themselves! In Vancouver, Canada, toddlers younger than two years old were given edible treats while their videotaped expressions of happiness were rated by two trained observers. The children were also asked to give treats to puppets that said YUMM. The greatest expressions of happiness were seen when the children gave their treats to the puppets.

So why is a preference for individuals who share goals so critical that nature ensures that we are born with it? Quite simply, cooperation (i.e., altruistic behaviors benefiting both recipient and actor) is the greatest tool in the human Swiss Army knife of survival. Acting together may start as a game, rolling the ball back and forth, but it snowballs to create our most common hallmarks of civilization. ABT is consonant with such ideas. Even if we don't *always* act accordingly, and act together, we all automatically intuit that we are "in this together." Thus, I think we can support the idea that the foundations of cooperation, kindness, and even altruism are intrinsic parts of the nerve cell biology of the human cerebral cortex.

The ability of very young children to behave in a caring, altruistic fashion strongly supports ABT. The fact that altruism is built in, that is, that we are wired for prosocial behavior in a manner analogous to our being wired to speak grammatically, allows even small children to exhibit the behavior. Indeed, if altruistic behaviors had to be learned by means of complex cognitive systems, children could not exhibit such behaviors. Thus the types of developmental studies carried out by scientists such as Tomasello and Wynn have yielded results that support the conclusion that the brain mechanisms for altruistic behaviors are straightforward, based on well-accepted neuroscience.

BROADER IMPLICATIONS: ABT'S CONNECTIONS TO RELIGION AND TO ETHICAL UNIVERSALITY

The explanation presented in Chapter 2 of the steps comprising ABT made no assumptions about special types of individuals capable of altruism. Such non-differentiation leads naturally to the idea that ABT is universal among humans. In fact, I first considered a neuroanatomical basis for altruistic action when I realized that there was a wide consensus around the idea that humans *should* behave in a reciprocally altruistic manner. Then I quickly discovered that such a consensus had a name, "moral universalism": the position that some system of ethics applies universally regardless of particular individuals' secondary distinguishing characteristics (e.g., race, sex, or religion). According to the philosopher R. W. Hepburn, such a view rests on the notion that "moral values exist independently of the feeling-states of individuals at particular times," that is, no matter how you feel about someone you must still behave toward him in a moral fashion. The linguist and political theorist Noam Chomsky goes further, not merely defining moral universalism but also arguing that it is basic to human relations:

> [W]e adopt the principle of universality: if an action is right (or wrong) for others, it is right (or wrong) for us. Those who do not rise to the minimal moral level of applying to themselves the standards they apply to others—more stringent ones, in fact— plainly cannot be taken seriously when they speak of appropriateness of response: or of right and wrong, good and evil.
>
> In fact, one of the, maybe the most, elementary of feature of moral principles is that of universality, that is, if something is right for me, it's right for you; if it's wrong for you, it's wrong for me. Any moral code that is even worth looking at has that at its core somehow.

Because so many religious and philosophical traditions seemed to cohere around the position of moral reciprocity, could there be a brain mechanism explaining such coherence? If there is such a mechanism, then we are all *equipped* to be good, and the overarching question becomes: how do we create conditions that favor our natural inclinations, and limit impulses that undermine such inclinations? This could be a game-changer, as we have so many institutions—courts, the diplomatic corps, prisons—that are premised on extreme wariness of presumed enemies and opponents, without stopping to calculate how such institutions might be reformed to accentuate the potential for decency even in the most depraved individuals.

Put another way, the idea of a natural proclivity toward moral reciprocity is important because it points to brain mechanisms that support civilization. Understanding altruism's hormonal and neural basis permits us to create circumstances conducive to civilization. The more you understand how something works (e.g., how the brain functions) the better you can arrange for it to work well, so that it does not break down so often. The implications for pharmacology, surgery, and social policy are obvious. If this seems far-fetched or something out of *1984*, consider how decoding the human genome—that is, the deepest structure of our genetic makeup—has spurred research into an array of potentially life-saving therapies. I am talking about the deep structure of the brain. Indeed, the point of all scientific data is to dispel myths and misconceptions about how humans can thrive in a challenging world, and understanding the brain is no different.

The point is that while ABT has finally shed scientific daylight on notions of morality, the pervasiveness of such notions—deeply ingrained in Western and non-Western cultures—sheds light on science's capacity to explain them. People have recognized for centuries that reciprocal morality exists, and they have been saying for centuries that we ought to practice it. Why such an outpouring unless there is some fundamental impulse—in effect, a wired-in ability—that accounts for it? This is not to say that a cultural norm "proves" science, but it does support a demonstration that biology underlies that set of precepts comprising the norm. Science and culture necessarily intersect. The brain is *responsible* for culture. Thus although it is true that scientists look for fundamental explanations unaffected by cultural or other exogenous factors, they also naturally see culture as an expression of the organ responsible for all behavior, the brain. Indeed, scientists have explained many social activities (e.g., cooperation) by examining the brain. But until recently, they have taken a back seat regarding moral reciprocity, leaving it to philosophers who do not so much explain as appreciate. Thus Simon Blackburn's *Ethics: A Very Short Introduction* states that requirements for reciprocal altruism can be "found in some form in almost every ethical tradition." The United Nations Declaration of Human Rights represents the political expression of such universality. My point is that though such cultural expressions of morality do not explain morality, they evoke a biological explanation of why they are so universal. They prompt a scientist to ask, as I did, how the norm originated in human biology.

CLASSICAL ORIGINS

While the neuroscience of ABT speaks for itself, it is interesting and reassuring to see how the coincidence of earlier views of morality implicitly pointed to the type of biological origin that ABT now supplies. I emphasize the universality of such views. In this regard, it would be difficult not to discuss the Greek philosopher Plato, among the first in recorded history to argue that a morally correct life is happier than an immoral one. First, he argued, because the desires of an immoral person are not constrained by morality, they expand past the point of possible satisfaction and lead to unhappiness. Second, he insisted that an immoral person must lack reason, and because reason gives rise to the greatest of human pleasures an immoral person would miss out on its joys. He concluded, therefore, that a morally correct life fosters a person's well-being, and was among the first to link morality with physicality, the "experience of pleasure"

By the 17th century, Baruch Spinoza argued that each human being is simply a finite part of Nature, maintaining by virtue of his behavior a balance with other humans and the rest of Nature. His ethics are premised on what "ought to be done," and contain an imperative toward moral reciprocity on which the very welfare of the world depends.

In the 18th century, the British philosopher David Hume tried to examine the means by which humans make moral judgments.

Specifically, he asked whether (on the one hand) morality requires intellectual calculation, a weighing of the pros and cons of benevolence, or (on the other hand) if it is more a "felt" affair, a decision that pulls on the heartstrings as well as the intellect. Seeking to explain the fact that humans do generally behave well, he decided against the prevailing view among many philosophers who extolled the power of our rational capacities. Instead, he came down on the side of what he called "moral sentiments."

Moral sentiments played a role in Hume's thinking similar to the role that "emotions" play in modern neuroscience. Echoing Plato, Hume argued that we derive pleasure and pride when we do something that is morally approved, but that we are discomfited and shamed when we do something that is not sanctioned. He then emphasized that reasoning alone could not motivate moral action. Rational thought, he explained, helps men figure out what is true and what is false, but is not helpful in judging right from wrong. For this latter distinction, we need to let our feelings guide us.

Statements amounting to the Golden Rule—that we should treat others as we would like to be treated ourselves—have been with us throughout history, across continents and centuries. This is the kind of behavioral disposition that, it is reasonable for a biological detective to suppose, might depend on discoverable brain mechanisms. The elucidation of ABT here has done the job.

SPEAKING TO A UNIVERSAL
ETHICAL PRINCIPLE

Apart from the classical philosophers, let's examine the evidence for a universal requirement for moral reciprocity. If you ask most religious leaders, they will say that the tenet that they all have in common is the Golden Rule in all its various expressions. In

1993, 143 leaders of the world's major faiths convened in Chicago to decide on what they called a Global Ethic, encompassing their religions' common principles. Delegates included respected representatives of Islam, Christianity, Judaism, Baha'i, Brahmanism, Brahma Kumaris, Taoism, Theosophism, Unitarian Universalism, and Zoroastrianism. They defined their own commonality as "We must treat others as we wish others to treat us." In effect, the Golden Rule. In the interest of advancing world peace and well-being, they issued a *Declaration Toward a Global Ethic*, embodying the Rule's sentiments:

> There is a principle which is found and has persisted in many religious and ethical traditions of humankind for thousands of years: What you do not wish done to yourself, do not do to others. Or in positive terms: What you wish done to yourself, do to others!...
>
> Every form of egoism should be rejected: All selfishness, whether individual or collective, whether in the form of class thinking, racism, nationalism, or sexism. We condemn these because they prevent humans from being authentically human. Self-determination and self-realization are thoroughly legitimate so long as they are not separated from human responsibility and global responsibility, that is, from responsibility for fellow humans and for planet Earth.

The *Declaration* does two things: it announces a requirement for moral reciprocity, and it acknowledges that such a requirement is sanctioned by time and across religious/ethical traditions. But it also goes further, stating that failure to live up to such a requirement would "prevent humans from being authentically human." Is moral reciprocity the *norm*, wired into the way our brains are constructed? That is, to be decent toward other humans is to be human in the most basic, physiological sense of that term.

Such reciprocity is useful to our survival, as it enables us to maintain a certain level of trust and expectation without which we could not function in a complex, highly networked society. To an extraordinary degree, the entire world economy depends on some version of the Golden Rule, calibrated to the needs of business. You think I'm exaggerating? Consider what was billed as "Global Ethics Summit 2012—Raising the Bar on Best Practices for Effective Corporate Ethics and Compliance," sponsored by Thomson Reuters and the Ethisphere Institute, with major financial support from the international law firm Hogan Lovells. The Summit's website proclaims:

> As companies continue to expand and compete in the global marketplace, they are met with constant reminders of the importance of maintaining global ethics an compliance program. The Global Ethics Summit will offer participants critical and timely insight into the risks and challenges of conducting business as well as best practices to mitigate the threats they pose.

Business people know that they need to rely on each other, even as they compete, because the "market" is actually a shared artifact where everyone creates an environment implicating everyone else—not just major buyers and sellers but also the everyday consumer. Without a certain level of ethical conduct leading to trust, business-to-business sales would collapse, as would transactions with consumers. In effect, there is a parallel ethical universality in business, resting on a requirement for reciprocally altruistic behavior that takes account of the circumstances of trade, a species of human relations. The difference, of course, is that outliers in business relations, that is, those who do not uphold ethical norms, are frequently punished. It is no accident that a representative of the U.S. Department of Justice was among the Summit's speakers.

Nor have businesspeople only recently come to realize that ethical behavior toward each other is crucial to their own viability. As far back as the 17th and 18th centuries, business manuals such as *The Trades-man's Calling* and *The Compleat English Tradesman* advocated ethical behavior among tradesmen on grounds that trade depended on trust. Cotton Mather, the great Protestant divine in Colonial America, proclaimed: "The Business of the CITY shall be managed by the Golden Rule," and "Were the Golden Rule generally regarded, there were need no Laws to force men to be Honest." As long-term credit became prevalent, and tradesmen began dealing with second—and third—parties whom they didn't know, the requirement became all the more important. As the market became increasingly complex, calls for honesty became louder. In *The Compleat English Tradesman* (1725–1727), perhaps the founding text in English with regard to the complex ethics of trade, Daniel Defoe observed that though some trading claims will always be vague or imperfect, honesty should be the goal.

Here are just a few of the many examples of historical evidence for Golden Rule–like prescriptions, demonstrating that they have been a feature of human relations for centuries. They all speak to a universal presence of Altruistic Brain operations in the human brain.

A papyrus from ancient Egypt, *c.* 664 B.C.E.–323 B.C.E., reads "That which you hate to be done to you, do not do to another." Similar examples from around the same period can be found among texts from ancient Greece.

Across the globe, in ancient China, Confucius states in the sacred *Analects*, written or compiled between 475 B.C.E. and 221 B.C.E., "Never impose on others what you would not choose for yourself." The sentiment is featured in the story of a disciple who asked for "one word which may serve as a rule of practice for all one's life?" Confucius answered "Is *reciprocity* not such a word? Do not to others what you do not want done to yourself—this is what the word means."

On the Indian subcontinent, we find such sentiments throughout influential epic tales and portions of the Vedic Scriptures, deemed Hinduism's oldest texts. From the *Mahabharata*, an Sanskrit epic regarded by some to have impacted world civilization with a weight comparative to the Bible and the Qur'ān, comes this quotation: "Do not to others what you do not wish done to yourself; and wish for others too what you desire and long for, for yourself—This is the whole of Dharma; heed it well."

While we are considering schools of thought arising from India, we must not overlook Buddhism, the fourth-largest religion in the world behind Christianity, Islam, and Hinduism. Like other great leaders, the historical Buddha Siddhartha Gautama, who taught in the 5th century B.C.E., made reciprocally altruistic behavior the keystone of his ethics. In the *Udanavarga* and elsewhere, he made the rule explicit: "Hurt not others in ways that you yourself would find hurtful" (Figure 5.1).

In view of current international concerns over Iran's nuclear ambitions, it is somewhat comforting, historically at least, to see that in an ancient but influential Iranian belief system, Zorastrianism, the prophet Zoroaster explained, "That which is good for all and any one, for whomsoever—that is good for me . . . . What I hold good for self, I should for all."

Of course, religious teachers are not alone in counseling ethical reciprocity. Consider, for example, Immanuel Kant's "categorical imperative," which states that one should consider each intended action as though it would dictate how every person should behave in a similar situation. Yet Kant is just one in a long line of philosophers drawing such conclusions. All of these religious leaders and philosophers were leaning toward ABT but it takes modern neuroscience to put it together.

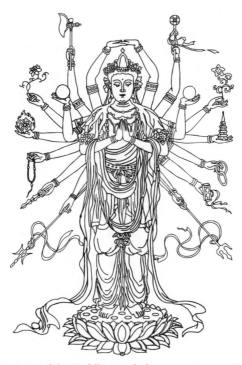

Figure 5.1 An image of the Buddha, symbolizing compassion. Many religions speak in sympathy with the principles of human behavior emanating from the Altruistic Brain. ABT finds its precedents.

PUTTING IT TOGETHER

The universality of statements reviewed in this chapter shows how ABT speaks to a widespread and continuing human need. It provides a compelling backdrop to the latest neuroscience research, and together they should help change our understanding of human altruism. As this book argues throughout, there is actually massive evidence to conclude that altruism is not just a "nice feature" of human behavior, but an innate capacity of our brains that meets a requirement for the maintenance of human society. *Homo sapiens'* brain is designed to support and enforce behaviors that help to *create* society and keep us from splaying off into isolated individual actors, unconcerned for the good of the whole.

In Chapter 6, we'll see how ABT can alter our view of ourselves and, indeed, of altruism.

FURTHER READING

Simon Blackburn. 2001. *Ethics: A Very Short Introduction*, p. 101. Oxford: Oxford University Press.

H. A. Chapman, D. A. Kim, J. M. Susskind, and A. K. Anderson. 2009. "In Bad Taste: Evidence for the Oral Origins of Moral Disgust." *Science* 323, 1222–1226.

Noam Chomsky. 2002. "Terror and Just Response," *ZNet*, July 2.

Richard Davidson and Anne Harrington, eds. 2002. *Visions of Compassion: Western Scientists and Tibetan Buddhists Examine Human Nature.* New York: Oxford University Press.

Daniel Defoe. 1725–1727. *The Compleat English Tradesman.*

Frans de Waal. 2006. *Primates and Philosophers.* Princeton, NJ: Princeton University Press.

Joshua Greene. 2005. "Cognitive Neuroscience and the Structure of the Moral Mind." In Peter Carruthers, Stephen Laurence, and Stephen Stich, eds., *The Innate Mind: Structure and Contents.* Oxford: Oxford University Press.

Joshua Greene, L. Nystrom, et al. 2004. "The Neural Bases of Cognitive Conflict and Control in Moral Judgment." *Neuron* 44, 389–400.

J. Kiley Hamlin, Karen Wynn, and Paul Bloom. 2010. "Three-Month-Olds Show a Negativity Bias in Their Social Evaluations." *Developmental Science* 1–7.

Thomas Hobbes. 1651. *Leviathan.*

Bert Hölldobler and Edward O. Wilson. 2008. *The Superorganism: The Beauty, Elegance, and Strangeness of Insect Societies.* New York: W. W. Norton.

David Hume. 1739. *Treatise of Human Nature.*

David Hume. 1777. *Enquiry Concerning the Principles of Morals.*

Immanuel Kant. 1785. *Foundations of the Metaphysics of Morals.*

John Locke. 1689. *The Second Treatise of Government.*

Andrew N. Meltzoff. 1995. "Understanding the Intentions of Others: Re-enactment of Intended Acts by 18-Month-Old Children." *Developmental Psychology* 31 838–850.

Steven Pinker. 2011. *The Better Angels of Our Nature: Why Violence Has Declined.* New York: Viking Penguin.

Hannes Rakoczy, Nina Brosche, Felix Warneken, and Michael Tomasello. 2009. "Young Children's Understanding of the Context-Relativity of Normative Games." *British Journal of Developmental Psychology* 27, 445–456.

D. Rand, J. Greene, and M. Nowak. 2012. "Spontaneous Giving and Calculated Greed." *Nature* 489, 427–430.

Paul Rozin and Edward B. Royzman. 2001. "Negativity Bias, Negativity Dominance, and Contagion." *Personality and Social Psychology Review* 5, 296–320.

Paul Rozin, Jonathan Haidt, and Katrina Fincher. 2009. "From Oral to Moral." *Science* 323, 1179–1180.

F. H. Marco Schmidt, Hannes Rakoczy, and Michael Tomasello. 2011. "Young Children Attribute Normativity to Novel Actions without Pedagogy or Normative Language." *Developmental Science* 14, 530–539.

F. H. Marco Schmidt and Jessica Sommerville. 2011. "Fairness Expectations and Altruistic Sharing in 15 Month-old Human Infants." *PLoS One* 6.10.

Simone Schnall, Jonathan Haidt, Gerald Clore, and Alexander Jordan. "Disgust as Embodied Moral Judgment." *Personality and Social Psychology Bulletin* 34, 1096–1109.

A. Shenhav and J. Greene. 2010. "Moral Judgments Recruit Domain-General Valuation Mechanisms to Integrate Representations of Probability and Magnitude." *Neuron* 67, 667–677.

Michael Tomasello. 2009. *Why We Cooperate*. Cambridge, MA: MIT Press.

Edward O. Wilson. 1978. *On Human Nature*. Cambridge, MA: Harvard University Press.

James Q. Wilson. 1993. *The Moral Sense*. New York: The Free Press.

PART II

IMPROVING PERFORMANCE OF THE MORAL BRAIN

Removing Obstacles to Good Behavior

[6]

HOW ALTRUISTIC BRAIN THEORY CHANGES OUR PERCEPTIONS OF OURSELVES AND OF ALTRUISM

Just as our neural wiring regulates everything we do, so everything we do reflects the operations of our brains. This includes not just autonomic and simple mechanical behaviors, but everything. The challenge to modern neuroscience, therefore, has become to go beyond the simple and to explain how the brain controls human behavior in complex social settings. So far, the friendliest social behaviors—for example, cooperation and parental nurturing—have proven relatively easy to explain, since we have evolved to favor such mutually supportive systems. I covered some of this work in Chapter 4.

In this chapter, however, I want to take this type of study to the next level: how our propensity for trust and cooperation can be stimulated, and called into play when people are arguing with each other. The question is a natural extension of now classic work on cooperation: what if, when people are angry or in situations that are naturally adversarial (for example, in a contract mediation proceeding) the brain's own capacities for altruism and mutuality could be made instrumental to settling the dispute? I argue that because we are wired to be mutually supportive, it is not enough merely to assert this fact and thank Evolution. Rather, we need to apply the best studies of our best behavior to real-life, troubling situations, so as to suggest how such studies can inform our social interactions when the going gets tough. Put another way, the next great challenge for behavioral neuroscience is to think about how complex, culturally inflected social situations can be understood—and potentially modified—in terms of the brain's own operations.

Right now, neuroscience is in its "golden age" as new, exciting techniques permit us to unravel how the brain regulates human behaviors of ever greater complexity. In their excitement, some neuroscientists may want to dismiss all previous approaches to how to regulate behavior. But they should not. Though it is true that today's techniques are unprecedented, the philosophical and religious evidence discussed previously in Chapter 5 is still worth taking into account insofar as it affirms basic human proclivities. Though there are sometimes radical discontinuities in science, known as "paradigm shifts," more often there is a slow accretion of knowledge that evolves from instinct to demonstration. Here we take a tiny step forward to apply Altruistic Brain Theory (ABT) to current attempts at improving self-image and cooperative behavior.

That is, all of the chapters will link ABT to current social problems, showing how it enhances our ability to approach those problems. In the spirit of the previous paragraph, I want to stress that ABT cannot "replace" the way we deal with issues; rather, it increases our understanding of how to deal with them given the tools that we have and will likely develop.

I have demonstrated so far that brain mechanisms have the effect of producing good, ethical, even altruistic behaviors. Now I will broach the operative question: so what? Assuming that our brains are wired for prosocial behavior, how does that affect the way we might organize our personal interactions to achieve a scaled social benefit? In succinct terms, if we can now—for the first time—really accept without dispute that we are naturally inclined toward empathy, what is the utility of such knowledge? Does it make the world function any better? If the potential for empathy has always been there, what is the incremental benefit of coming into an awareness of that potential? Now that we understand that altruistic acts are an inevitable consequence of very ordinary mechanisms in our brains, I'll describe new research that showing such understanding feeds back onto our ideas of ourselves.

Most importantly, the certainty that our brains work to produce moral behavior has vast and immediate consequences, starting with the power of self-image to influence individual behavior. The way that we view ourselves and each other is crucial to our social interactions. Thus if we know with certainty that we can tap into our own and others' altruistic capacities, then we can work toward transcending obstacles that prevent our giving effect to those capacities. On at least a small scale—even if only one-on-one—we can proceed with enhanced trust in ourselves and in those with whom we interact. Once focused on a goal involving trust in ourselves and each other, we will be less likely to give up and more likely to envision the morally preferable act and carry it out.

Think about that for a moment. Adolescents give into negative peer pressure because they lack confidence in their own best instincts. But if they could be assured of their natural prosocial potential, they might have greater ability to resist peer pressure; with Wesley Autrey, they could just "do the right thing."

THE EFFECT OF INDIVIDUAL SELF-IMAGE ON INDIVIDUALS' CAPACITY TO SUCCEED

Numerous studies have demonstrated that how we view ourselves has a direct effect on how we view, and hence interact with, other people. A social worker in the South Bronx told me that she has "a ton of examples and stories" in which she witnessed how someone's self-image as a good and effective person can influence his or her subsequent behavior. In one example, a student fell under the wrong influences as a young child. He had no feeling of self-worth, got in with the wrong crowd, and began getting into trouble, including robbing stores. He was arrested at 15 and was in jail for 6 months. When he was released, he got into a behavior-changing program that convinced him that he could have "life after incarceration," and that he actually had possibilities. He began to see himself in a different life, and as able to be useful. He earned a GED degree and has been functioning well for four years, including holding a job.

A person's positive self-image thus influences his individual social behavior, and, as it turns out, a positive self-image can support increased intellectual achievement. Carol Dweck and her team at Stanford have repeatedly demonstrated that when children believe that their traits are fixed, their performance is adversely affected, whereas if they are taught that their mental abilities are like muscles and can be made stronger with effort, they seek opportunities to learn and respond to setbacks with renewed effort and persistence. In one of Dweck's studies, seventh graders' beliefs that "intelligence is malleable," and able to be improved through continued effort, predicted an upward trajectory during two years of junior high school; students who believed that intelligence is fixed, however, had a flat trajectory. In a study dealing with self-control, people who felt that their ability to control eating was not fixed were able to limit what they ate under difficult conditions. In Dweck's words, " . . . reduced self-control after a depleting task or during demanding periods may reflect people's beliefs about the availability of (*their own*) willpower." Thus people's assessments of their own capacities—moral or intellectual—can influence their achievements, in school or in society. These kinds of data reinforce my argument that people who accept their own Altruistic Brain wiring can be expected to behave with greater altruism and trust.

The scientific basis for the social worker's story, as well as for the phenomena that Carol Dweck reported, is well-established in the principle of cognitive dissonance. Cognitive dissonance theory, which has gathered a tremendous amount of scholarly support over the decades, was introduced in 1957 by the Stanford psychology professor Leon Festinger. The principle states that people behave in ways that reduce the psychological distance between a belief that they hold and an intended action. Thus if someone truly believes that Ford is better than Chevrolet, not only will he buy the Ford, but he will also pay less attention to Chevy ads and more to those of Ford *so that his belief system can remain intact.* The principle has been used to increase use of condoms, reduce littering, reduce racial prejudice, and help regulate weight and diet. So in our case, if a young boy has been educated to believe that his brain has the intrinsic capacity to support his role as a good person, he will think of himself as good and will tend to act as a good person would act. Faced with temptation, he will tend to avoid it. In sum, our concept of our self influences our subsequent social behavior.

In this vein, Dan Ariely, professor of behavioral economics at Duke, explored the phenomenon of "the pot calling the kettle black." Sometimes, as Ariely says, "people are guilty of the very thought they identify in others." To reduce "ethical dissonance," they judge others more harshly, and at the same time "present themselves as more virtuous and ethical." Regarding the neural basis of the "dark side," the negative form of the cognitive dissonance principle, neuroscientists have begun to explore the brain mechanisms associated with low self-esteem. Low self-esteem, produced for example by early-life abuse and neglect, correlates with an excess secretion of stress hormones from the adrenal gland, particularly in response to a difficult situation. These hormones, as shown by Bruce McEwen of Rockefeller University, have particularly strong effects on a crucial part of the brain involved in both cognitive and emotional behavior: the hippocampus. Thus it is striking that a group of scientists at

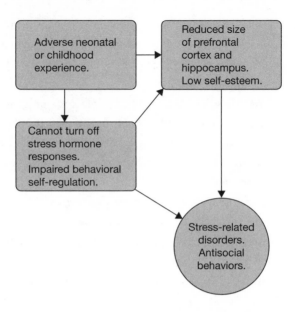

Figure 6.1 The results of Rockefeller University professor Bruce McEwen and others have charted the neurobiological and behavioral consequences of adverse neonatal or childhood experiences (left page) with those following nurturant early experiences (right page).

McGill University have shown that low self-esteem was associated with a shrunken hippocampus. Furthermore, psychiatric researchers at Harvard University connected childhood mistreatment with a reduced volume of the hippocampus. As a result of these studies, I believe that in a mistreated young boy, low self-esteem leads to antisocial behaviors, at least in part because of the effects of excess stress hormones acting in the brain, especially in the hippocampus. Good self-esteem—stemming from the knowledge that our brains are wired to be good—could have important effects on how young people behave (Figure 6.1).

As a corollary to the foregoing, low self-esteem affects how we are perceived by others and how we think other people should treat

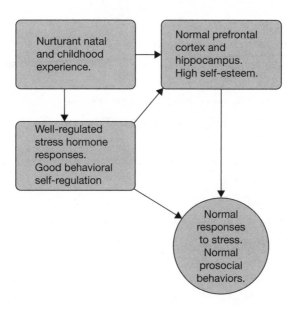

Figure 6.1 Continued

us. A sense of self-worth makes it possible for us to volunteer, join communal efforts, and expect to be treated fairly. Other people pick up on our sense of self, such that lacking a sense of self-worth can be a source of peril. Consider this statement in the Sunday Observer column of the *New York Times* (April 15, 2012), relating to the shooting of a black teen-ager, Trayvon Martin, by a Hispanic on neighborhood-watch patrol in a Florida suburb:

> Young black men know that in far too many settings they will be seen not as individuals, but as the "other," and given no benefit of the doubt. By the time they have grown into adult bodies—even though they are still children—they are well-versed in the experience of being treated as criminals until proved otherwise by the cops who stop and search them and eyed warily by nighttime pedestrians who cower on the sidewalks.

Society's message to black boys—"we fear you and view you as dangerous"—is constantly reinforced. Boys who are seduced by this version of themselves end up on a fast track to prison and to the graveyard. But even those who keep their distance from this deadly idea are at risk of losing their lives to it. The death of Trayvon Martin vividly underscores that danger.

One prong of this stark analysis—framed in terms of black men but applicable to everyone—is that assumptions that we make about people, especially whole classes of people, are invariably internalized by those people, often with horrible consequences. The analysis suggests that such assumptions can be "seductive," that they acquire the perverse appeal of a type of truth that becomes irresistible. Where people have not acquired a strong sense of self that would allow them to resist such public branding, perhaps because they have always suffered from society's indifference, they grasp at even the meanest "version of themselves" if it can fill the void. In effect, such people become the thing that others project onto them, sacrificing whatever capacity they may retain to function in society and accept social norms. Studies have demonstrated this syndrome in several cases.

If on the other hand we are convinced, through ABT and other sources, of our capacity for decent behavior, we will be more readily accepted, and will have the confidence to follow through. *Understanding that we have an inherent proclivity to be good is therefore useful.* Here are three examples of how, in light of ABT, I can suggest applications of the theory to current problems in human behavior.

1. *Resisting negative peer pressure.* Studies of adolescents have shown that they are highly vulnerable to negative peer pressure. They join gangs; they smoke; they do drugs. In large measure, this is because they want to belong to a group that they imagine enhances their individual status and provides affirmation by virtue of a collective sameness. Yet what if teenagers at risk could be given a firm sense

that they were "better than that," that they possessed a capacity for moral behavior that was in itself commendable, and was a foundation for personal and social value irrespective of others' affirmation? To understand that one is good—when this is new information—is immensely liberating, freeing one from the need to seek approval beyond the circumference of a personal moral compass. Though students are taught "self-esteem" early in their careers, this is often a generalized feel-good therapy that results in reduced aspiration. If instead (or at least in addition) they were taught to understand and appreciate their inherent capacity for kindness, decency, and even altruism, they might be better equipped to face down negative pressures. A kid could simply say "I'm good and I know it," that is, my brain naturally and instinctively produces my good behavior; any other type of behavior would seem unnatural and self-defeating.

2. *Encouraging empathy.* A recent movement in schools around the world has been sparked by efforts to encourage empathy even in the lowest grades. One organization, Roots of Empathy, has developed an extensive program enabling students to develop empathy and apply it in real-life settings. Another group, the Collaborative for Academic, Social, and Emotional Learning, has similar if broader goals, teaching children how to master "relationship" skills. Such efforts are in sync with attempts by progressive educators to promote social and emotional development, and to help rescue children on the brink of emotional withdrawal. Teachers model empathic behaviors and seek to engender respect in peer-to-peer relationships. They direct children to others' critical emotional needs and encourage a type of perspective-taking through which the children can stand in those others' shoes. Indeed, Roots of Empathy offers a comprehensive nine-month program in which children can become emotionally attached to a baby: they hold her, sing to her, and create a "wishing tree" for the baby's future. Throughout the program, skilled instructors with detailed lesson plans guide the children in evaluating and

learning from their own and others' emotional responses. Studies have shown that where children go through these programs, they emerge as better behaved and, hence, more likely to succeed academically.

Mary Gordon, the founder of Roots of Empathy, argues that the capacity for empathy is "innate," "already there," and that we can create circumstances in which children—even damaged children—can "pull empathy out of themselves" where it has been buried on account of disuse. In her program, children become partners in the "construction" of empathic relationships, rather than objects of "instruction" that might be expected to absorb ideas about empathy based on what they are taught. She believes that by experiencing empathy, children come to an awareness of their own capacity for connection and relationship, that they achieve "a cognitive experience by means of by means of an emotional experience."

When we asked Gordon how an understanding of ABT supported her approach, she responded that it provided scientific proof for what she already knew from her 16 years' work with Roots of Empathy. "I never doubted that empathy was inborn." She went on to suggest that, clearly, empathy is "universal," not situational, and as applicable to children in a classroom as it is to enemies in Gaza. That is, anyone can display it toward anyone. So my question is: how can we build on Gordon's realization? How can neuroscience deepen children's sense that empathy is part of the natural order?

In my view, children should be enabled to experience and accept their own as well as others' empathetic inclinations in an *array* of settings that make such experiences appear grounded in basic human nature. Empathy should never be presented as a local, conditional response, but as a structural component of human nature.

Children should be put in circumstances where they can *discover* this fact for themselves. They should learn it in science classes, perhaps in a unit on the mammalian brain. We could depict for students the actual brain mechanisms behind empathy, so that it does not seem like just another emotion but, rather, like a built-in capacity of their own and others' mentality. Numerous teaching philosophies are based on children's discovering the natural world for themselves and so I suggest that we add encounters with empathy to this list. Empathy, though a building block of "social relations," is at its most basic a scientific principle that we can *understand*. The point is that we will be more inclined to practice empathy if we appreciate that it is intrinsic to how, as humans, we have literally been designed. It's not just that we "are" empathetic (having learned that this is a valued trait), but that we can be certain that we *evolved* to function as empathetic beings. Evolution itself can be taught in terms of the basic human traits with which it has endowed us.

Encouraging empathy can be effective even in very young children. The Harvard professor of developmental psychologist Elizabeth Spelke has reported that reciprocal behavior patterns can be displayed by children as young as three years of age. Indeed, even younger children exhibit the capacity for empathy; at 14 months they help others attain their goals. Developmental psychologist Michael Tomasello performed studies in which the experimenter was using clothespins to hang towels on a line, "accidentally" dropped a clothespin on the floor, and unsuccessfully reached for it. The infant helped by picking up the clothespin and handing it to the experimenter. In another situation, the experimenter was trying to put a sack of magazines into a cabinet but could not open the doors because his hands were full. The child helped by opening the door for him. Clearly, Altruistic Brain circuitry develops very early. The point is to design strategies to elicit this capacity effectively, rather than to start from the assumption that it must be taught from scratch. Such strategies might demonstrate to children that they naturally respond to another's need virtually without thinking, and that others respond to theirs in the same manner. Once children come to believe in their own capacities, they will retain that belief, literally without further coaxing.

But once taught, how does empathy "take hold?" How do temporary events in a child's life affect behavior for years to come? The scientific answer to this question is important, because as psychologists such as Mary Rothbart and Jerome Kagan have explained, once epochal experiences have affected one's temperament, this temperament will inflect all of one's social and emotional behaviors. There are times early in children's lives when one event—or many—can affect their temperaments forever, especially if such events are unfortunate. Scientists have wondered: what physical changes in the brain constitute the emotional "memory" by which behavior is altered, perhaps over the rest of one's life? One such suggested mechanism involves changes in the synapses (connections) between neurons. But a newly recognized mechanism is more convincing, and makes use of recent applications of molecular biology to neuroscience. These are the so-called "epigenetic" effects of early experience that I will now use to explain some aspects of temperament formation.

Specifically, remember that "epigenetics" refers to changes in gene functions—that is, changes that govern gene expression for a very long time—without requiring any mutation in the DNA sequence itself. Those "epigenetic" effects could occur in proteins in the nerve cell nucleus that cover the cell's DNA; they could be due to other chemicals in the cell nucleus; and they could occur by chemical decorations on individual parts of the DNA chain. Any or all of these could work. The consequences are enormous because they affect the brain and last a long time (Figure 6.2).

For example, suppose these epigenetic changes happen in neurons that produce serotonin, the neurotransmitter crucial to emotions, or in neurons that respond to serotonin. Trevor Robbins found that boosting serotonin effects in the synapses between neurons caused subjects "to judge harmful actions as forbidden, but only in cases where harms were emotionally salient." Serotonin "promoted prosocial behavior by enhancing harm aversion." This kind

Old View

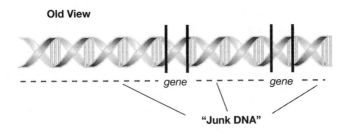

New View

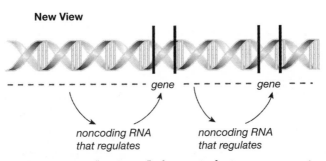

Figure 6.2 Long-term, "epigenetic" changes in brain gene expression can depend on noncoding RNAs that derive from DNA formerly called "junk DNA."

of neurochemical change gets translated into long-term changes in behavior by the construction of what the Japanese neuroscientist Atsushi Iriki calls "neuronal niches." Iriki envisions that neural circuits will be created to have stable performances that promote prosocial behavior. Creation of such "neural niches" allows transitory events, such as training in empathic behavior, to be turned into temperamental traits. The result can influence the functioning of important regions of the brain. For example, when Richard Davidson's lab at the University of Wisconsin studied brain activity in Buddhist monks trained in a form of meditation involving compassion, a functional magnetic resonance imaging (fMRI) scan lit up "a sprawling (brain) circuit that switches on at the sight of suffering." ABT tells us that once the "suffering circuit" is lit up, the normal individual will rapidly and automatically avoid the harmful behavior that caused it to light up. In this respect, Richard Davidson's result transports moral compassion into the domain of "neural plasticity"—the changeability and indeed the improvability of the human brain—established firmly by neuroscience pioneers such as Eric Kandel at Columbia Medical School, who studied much different types of neuronal systems.

THE EFFECT OF EMPATHY ON RELATIONSHIP FORMATION

The foregoing examples discuss the effect of understanding one's capacity for goodness on one's ability to succeed. The following examples examine the effect of understanding *others'* capacity for goodness, an inevitable consequence of ABT, on one's own ability to form relationships. Relationships depend on trust, and the basis for trust—apart from knowing that the State will enforce its laws—is our sense that someone has values more or less like our own. I will argue that understanding the universality of altruistic impulses, such that they are natural not just to us personally but to everyone, is crucial to establishing trust and to forming relationships of all kinds.

1. *Personal relationships, the central role of trust.* Many people have difficulty establishing trust. Hence they have difficulty with intimacy and relationships. One application of ABT is that if people could be persuaded of others' inherent decency, they might be better able to open up toward and then trust them. This could be a useful approach to healing and to enabling people to succeed at relationship formation. What is the nature of "trust?" It is seeing something of oneself in another, such that we can relax, feel comfortable, and *anticipate* that what we say will be understood. Without being able to take for granted some level of comprehension and empathy on the part

of another, we withdraw, we do not speak at all except insofar as we remain protective of ourselves. The ability to let go of such protective reticence, and to speak openly and candidly about what matters to us, emanates from trust and is crucial to relationship formation. The ABT demonstrates, even to people who are skeptical of others, that there is ground for hope, that is, hope that other people are not merely opportunists and egocentrics but rather available—like us— to engage in intimacy. For those people who have been harmed as youngsters, whether by parents, intimates, or perhaps abusive clergy, there is a chance once again to see human beings in a light favorable to establishing trust.

Needless to say, establishing trust in a relationship takes practice and affirmation; blind trust is naïve. Nevertheless, if we can teach people that they share a common decency, and that lapses from such commonality that they encountered were aberrations, then we have reinforced the ability to trust. An important part of counseling strategy, therefore, is to present the case that people are by nature prosocial, and that the possibility of relationship is not out of the question. Healing begins to take place when an individual is willing to consider the evidence, and to apply it going forward.

2. *Relationships in a broader social context.* Moreover, lest some think that "trust" is a fuzzy notion, okay for intimate personal relationships but hardly the stuff of hardnosed public policy, they need to think again. Recent scholarship points to the benefits of reincorporating notions of mutual trust into the nation's political, economic, and legal institutions. This is ABT placed on "a big stage," that of business and politics.

In all three areas, Professor Russell G. Pearce of Fordham Law School and Professor Eli Wald of the University of Denver Sturm College of Law have explained the importance and desirability of promoting reciprocal relationships. They note that the belief that people and organizations are atomistic or autonomous has undermined many modern relationships, cultures, and institutions. From this perspective, people and organizations understand the concept of "self-interest" as maximizing short-term and narrow self-interest, without regard for how their conduct impacts others and their community. Pearce and Wald argue that a more realistic—and beneficial—understanding is that people and organizations exist relationally and therefore that the self-interest of individuals or organizations is inevitably connected to the self-interest of their neighbors and communities.

Pearce and Wald apply this analysis to the seemingly intractable incivility that dominates modern American political culture. "Harsh" and "vitriolic" political rhetoric relies on the assumption that politics is a "zero sum" competition between atomistic individuals and groups. The prevalence of this behavioral assumption dooms efforts to promote civility by making moral arguments for civility appear naïve and unpersuasive. In addition, proposals to counter civility with centrist politics will not make any difference to the behavioral assumptions that promote incivility, even if they succeed in promoting a centrist political agenda.

A way to restore civility to political debate is to shift the behavioral assumptions of the relevant actors. If political actors were to take on board Altruistic Brain insights and incorporate them into their discourse, they could create a political culture that promoted prosocial behavior and discouraged incivility. Social interaction is not a zero sum game, whether on the personal or political level. Political actors would be better off in a system where the benefits of reciprocity and cooperation were a given. If we ignore this approach, we risk a perpetual cycle of aggressive, antisocial discourse that hampers any possibility of compromise.

Pearce and Wald offer the example of Martin Luther King, Jr. Although he faced "mobs of angry, hate-filled, and sometimes violent white people committed to denying black people their fundamental human rights," King urged his followers "to attack the evil system rather than the individuals who happen to be caught up in the system." They should not "aim...to defeat the white community, not to humiliate the white community, but to win the friendship of all of the persons who had perpetrated this system in the past." Rejecting the notion of politics as a "zero-sum game," he pursued "reconciliation and the creation of a beloved community." King's approach accords with the understanding of ABT.

As Pearce and Wald also observe, Nobel Prize winner Amartya Sen and other leading economists have long turned to approaches that emphasize reciprocity. For example, economists Luigino Bruni and Robert Sugden identify a weakness in prevailing economic theories grounded in the belief that maximizing narrow self-interest is the only motivation of economic actors.

They point out that such theories fail to account for the way people generally do not take advantage of each other when contracts are invalid and or when one party to a contract requires an adjustment to avoid a significant loss. Instead, Bruni and Sugden explain that mutual benefit offers a better description of economic behavior. People and organizations seek to benefit themselves, but they also prefer economic exchanges (and social relationships) that benefit both their self-interest and that of others.

ABT provides a powerful argument for this understanding and a powerful explanation for why contrary strategies cause harm. Bruni and Sugden note one example. Where there is no trust, parties are less likely to enter into economic exchanges and create economic value. The Great Recession offers another example of the effects of a decline in relational self-interest. Society suffered—and continues to suffer—extensive damage from economic behavior that ignored relational self-interest in favor of the narcissistic appeal of seeking short-term gains without concern for harms to others. Indeed, under Bruni and Sugden's analysis, ABT becomes a tool for a healthy capitalist economy.

Relational approaches to politics and economics make sense under ABT. But how would society move toward this goal? One way, of course, is for people to come to understand the dynamic of moral reciprocity and commit themselves to acting accordingly. This chapter offers grounds for doing so. Indeed, Pearce and Wald assert that "we must begin to organize social institutions to avoid undermining and to promote reciprocal relationships to take advantage of" our capacities for reciprocal altruism.

They offer two examples of how to do this. The first is changing our approach to government regulation of businesses. Today, the common approach to regulation is "command and control." It assumes that regulated individuals and entities care only about their autonomous self-interest. Command and control regulations tell people what to do and penalize them if they fail to comply. But when the government assumes that actors care only about their narrow self-interest, it reinforces the regulated parties' beliefs that their self-interest requires them to do whatever they can get away with inside the bounds of the law. This ethos, in turn, leads them to seek strategies that will allow them to pursue their antisocial goals without transgressing the letter of a particular law, and requires the government in turn to develop new regulations to prohibit this newly discovered antisocial conduct, in a never-ending cycle.

Many scholars recommend that the government instead pursue what are called principles—or outcome-based regulatory strategies. Under these approaches, the government prescribes the general outcomes it seeks from regulated parties, which then have the responsibility for preparing their own plan for achieving these objectives. They submit their plan to the government and enter a dialogue regarding whether their plan adequately addresses the government's goals.

This regulatory strategy promotes reciprocal relationships. Rather than view itself as an adversary of the government, the regulated entity understands the relationship as reciprocal. The entity and the government work together on creating the final product based on a proposal that the entity itself has developed. Within the entity, moreover, employees work together to consider how the proposed regulations ought to be implemented. This cooperative effort makes them more likely to understand themselves and their organization as having a reciprocal relationship with each other, the government, and those whom the regulations seek to protect.

Command and control models not only reflect the cultural dominance of autonomous self-interest, but also shape and help constitute it. Outcome-based approaches encourage, incentivize, and empower a more relational understanding of self and others.

Pearce and Wald's second recommendation is that the legal system itself better promote reciprocal relationships. They note that since the 1960s most lawyers have followed a hired gun ideal that seeks to maximize the autonomous self-interest of themselves and their clients. Given this mentality, approaches that seek to promote cooperative resolution of conflicts are described as "alternative" dispute resolution. But Pearce and Wald argue that given the importance of law and the central role it plays in terms of structuring relationship, lawyers should encourage clients to pursue their relational self-interest. If they were to do so, reconciliation rather than adversity could become a central, although not the exclusive goal of the legal system—certainly not peripheral or "alternative." When we discuss alternative dispute resolution, in the text that follows, we examine it from this perspective.

We live in a legal environment that does not provide incentives for reciprocal relationships, as the general American law is that a person has no obligation to help someone in dire need. This approach, different than that found in most countries, codifies the idea that we have no obligations to each other. A different set of rules—often known as Good Samaritan laws—would encourage us to provide reasonable aid to a neighbor in peril, providing a measure of legal protection as an incentive.

Needless to say, all of these initiatives to bring ABT to bear on political, economic, and legal culture will meet resistance. Yet there is good reason to accommodate settled practice to what we now know concerning human nature. Because we know that moral reciprocity is humanity's default position and we believe it is desirable, it would seem incumbent on us to work to develop institutions and cultures that foster moral reciprocity. If we are wired to favor reciprocity and prosocial behaviors, then these approaches should eventually bear fruit.

Moreover, even where economic, political, and legal actors do not recognize the full potential of reciprocal relationships, many successful people have built their careers to some extent on reciprocal relationships, whether the banker who had a mentor, a small businessperson who is a pillar of the community and in turn receives that community's support, a law partner who cultivates a recurring retainer with a prized client, or a politician who appreciates the importance of trusting relationships with ideological allies.

ABT provides the foundation for, and explains the potential for expanding, these understandings in ways that benefit our society and each other. After all, if it is natural and desirable to support one another, then shouldn't the economic, political, and legal culture promote—and not discourage—this result?

3. *The effect of empathy in alternative dispute resolution.* A thorough understanding of ABT should render alternative dispute resolution (ADR) proceedings more likely to succeed. This is because participants' knowledge of each other's Golden Rule circuitry will facilitate the trust that ADR depends on.

Indeed, clearing the way to successful ADR proceedings is important to this country's administration of justice. With federal and state court dockets backed up literally for years, and an accompanying shortage of judges, potential litigants are turning to ADR in increasing numbers. Without many of the formal constraints of the judicial system, ADR offers a means to settle even complex disputes more quickly and with less expense. The question, however, is how ADR can be made to work optimally, so that it offers not just a default, but a desirable "alternative" to the litigation process. After examining techniques employed by ADR practitioners, I think that perhaps ABT has a part to play in addressing this concern. Such practitioners agree that as in personal relationships ADR's success pivots on the establishment of trust. Unlike in court proceedings, individuals who embark on ADR need to find common ground to work out their differences and find a resolution. Citing ABT as grounds for trust, ADR facilitators can encourage these individuals to trust each other's motives—both are seeking a fair resolution. They can remind even the most vehemently opposed individuals that their natural inclinations are good and, despite the current disagreement, they have the *capacity* to empathize with and trust one another, if only they could acknowledge each other's decency. At the very least, facilitators can remind opponents that they share a goal, literally "dispute resolution," and that there is reason to trust each other because both parties want to reach this goal, rather than allow the whole process to collapse. Trust can be built into the resolution process as a practical component that will move the process along.

The Conflict Research Consortium of the University of Colorado recently published an article citing the fundamental role of empathy in establishing trust, and hence in moving the resolution process forward: "Mediators can help the parties establish trust and work together effectively...Allowing all the parties to 'tell their stories'— to explain how they feel and why—can generate a level of understanding and empathy that begins to break down barriers between people." Empathy is not just a feel-good modality so that people do not shout at each other or perceive one another as threats. It is instrumental, allowing people to achieve some level of trust, crucial to the success of the resolution process. Telling one's story ("I would have paid my rent but I lost my job and got sick") is humanizing and can testify to character. If it leads to trust, the parties will learn still more about each other and the nature of their dispute. Writing in *Beyond Intractability*, the negotiator Richard Salem, who served on the initial training committee of South Africa's National Peace Accord, observed that "When trust levels are high, parties are less defensive and more willing to share information with other parties at the mediation table and in private sessions with the mediator—information that may be crucial to finding a mutually acceptable solution." It is hardly a new idea, therefore, to stress the importance of empathy in dispute resolution, and to link it to the establishment of trust; what neuroscience offers is another, extremely persuasive ground for impressing the parties that empathy is both possible and "normal." It is everyone's default condition, which should be encouraged at the outset (and during the progress) of an ADR proceeding so as to promote the proceeding's success.

The role of trust-building between the parties is crucial and, in fact, there is a vast academic literature on how trust is established. D. Harrison McKnight and Norman L. Chervany observe in an important piece entitled "Reflections on an Initial Trust-Building Model" that "Like water, the need for trust is not noticed until it becomes scarce in an environment." That is, as we embark on new relationships—indeed, new types of relationships—we look for ways to make those relationships cohere. I will come back to the literature on trust again, but I want to emphasize here that there would be no academic percentage in investigating trust—no possibility of grants, publications, or tenure—if the subject were merely speculative, a type of metaphysics. Trust is necessary for the world to work properly. Anything that we can do to create it will have major consequences.

As already suggested, when the parties to a proceeding communicate, each can recognize elements in the other that are reassuring, that demonstrate in effect that one party is as capable of good will as the other. The conversation does not even have to be face-to-face, as online dispute resolution is now an integral part of e-commerce, resolving millions of disputes a year. One of the leading practitioners in the area is Colin Rule, a Fellow of Stanford's Center for Internet and Society, CEO of Modria (an online dispute resolution service), and the first director of dispute resolution at Pay-Pal and eBay. As Rule told us:

> Much of dispute resolution is based on the concept that people want to do the right thing, and that direct and honest communication can enable people to get past the misconceptions that lead us to mistreat each other. We confuse ourselves into thinking we need to be pushy and impolite to others to get them to act fairly, [because] I've seen hundreds of cases where people talk with each other, clear up those misconceptions, and reach agreement. I know thousands of my fellow dispute resolvers have the same experience every day. That's proof that at base we are wired to cooperate.

What's interesting here is that Rule is speaking from inside capitalism, where what matters is that transactions keep humming and not get hung up on remote parties' disagreements. Rule's point is that in an environment of absolutely zero sentimentality—nobody knows you, nobody's looking out for you—trust is still the operative principle. He describes the limit case, yet still concludes that we are "wired" to cooperate. I will examine such remote relationships in detail later, but for now it's useful to observe that if trust can so easily surface—and be relied on—in e-commerce exchanges, then how much more likely is it that trust can be operative in the face-to-face context of ADR? Indeed, in an article aptly entitled "Trust breaks down in electronic contexts but can be repaired by some initial face-to-face contact," Elena Rocco demonstrates that where electronic contacts get off to a shaky start, some follow-up conversation can ensure a successful experience. The *capacity* for trust is always present and can be restored, because even where our interests are opposed we still respond to each other's humanity and fall into patterns of trust.

Such recognition is universal and transcendent, while the opposition is particular and temporal. Given such universality—that is, given that we are naturally inclined to empathize and, hence, develop trust—I think that ADR proceedings should take the potential for trust to the next level. Some process for *fostering* mutual recognition should be institutionalized, so that ADR proceedings would routinely start by establishing plausible grounds for trust. Perhaps such grounds could develop from an exchange of biographies, in which life-changing common experiences—a divorce, a hysterectomy—could be shared. Perhaps both parties were in the Marines. Perhaps they would simply understand that there doesn't *need* to be an affinity because science now knows that we are wired to empathize. In any case, the point is that because the parties are naturally inclined toward empathy, then that empathy should be brought to the fore in advance, making it easier for the parties to achieve a level of trust sufficient to reach a fair settlement. As I mentioned earlier, the facilitator could start by encouraging parties to trust each other's honest desire to reach some resolution that both parties can live with, and that minimizes the time, money, and pain that each has to invest in reaching that resolution. As Rule notes, even though trust initially requires "a leap of faith," communities have both the interest and capacity to foster trust.

4. *Conflict resolution proceedings.* Conflict resolution is akin to ADR but more broadly focused, and is not necessarily a surrogate for litigation. It also depends on the kind of trust that ABT encourages.

Conflict resolution addresses disputes of more or less any kind, for example, collective bargaining, and even those between parties from different countries and subject to different legal traditions. The Center for the Study of Narrative and Conflict Resolution at George Mason University, in Virginia, is one of the leading examples of how the whole area of conflict resolution is being brought into a productive relationship with an array of academic disciplines, all of which add theoretical heft to the delivery of conflict resolution services. The Center's mission statement points to the centrality of conversation, give-and-take, and what it calls the role of "narrative" in the resolution process, and in this regard it provides an opening for precisely the type of trust that can be fostered and utilized in drawing parties toward agreement:

> Conflict is the discursive process in which people struggle for legitimacy, caught in stories they did not make (by themselves) and all too often, cannot change—the network of social relationships, histories, and institutional processes restrict the nature of stories that can be told. Conflict, for this perspective, is a narrative process in which the creation, reproduction and transformation of meaning itself is a political process—a struggle against marginalization and delegitimization, for legitimacy, if not hegemony. Narratives matter.

The statement suggests that within the frame of the resolution process, the parties "struggle" over meaning and legitimacy but do not necessarily emerge as Winners or Losers. Meaning is created and transformed in a kaleidoscopic telling of the facts...until at some point it is settled sufficiently for each party to accept that version of how the conflict should play out. "Narratives matter," according to the statement, because narrative is the vehicle by which settlement is reached. I would argue, therefore, that without faith in the narrative as it develops, the parties will just give up and go home, fighting again in some other arena at another time. To establish such faith—that is, trust in the ongoing narrative—the parties must be able to trust one another. Because they may not even know each other, the facilitator in charge of the proceedings could introduce them to ABT.

On the other hand, of course, they may know each other all too well. Think, for example, of a divorce proceeding. Here, where love and even goodwill may have almost completely broken down, one might argue that the parties are simply too angry with one another to even think about empathy—much less feel and express it. Trust is simply unthinkable! Yet *even* in the case of divorce, there is a possibility for some trust to develop. If both parties come to the table understanding that they share a common interest in minimizing costly, protracted fighting, and that each can be trusted insofar as they will both work toward that end, then minimal common ground can be established from which to make a start. The point is to *start* working together, and then build on that. Studies have shown that once people (even enemies) start working together, and experience a mutual capacity for cooperation, trust grows. ABT is useful to get people to the table, that is, to convince them that it is worth making assumptions about the possibility of redeveloping a working collaboration based on empathy and trust, *even though both those feelings have collapsed.* They can begin to view empathy and trust as in their own best interests, as utilitarian modalities that will make the path to their shared goal that much easier to tread. An analogous argument could be made with regard to marriage counseling, where many of the same issues are at stake.

One could, of course, imagine all sorts of settings in which the goal is simply to work out a *modus vivendi*, literally a means of living within a situation so that the fighting stops and people get on with their lives. At its core, this is what conflict resolution is about, as everyone is way too busy to indulge in protracted argument (the Crusades had a certain glamor, but don't expect them to resume under capitalism). In this regard, I would like to cite Colin Rule again, who described his experience at the dawn of big-time e-commerce when eBay was trying to formulate rules for organizing online trades, and was also anticipating the volume of disputes that might conceivably gum up the works. Presciently, the company started from the premise that people should be able to trust one another:

> Pierre Omidyar drafted a set of values for eBay when he first started the site in the mid-1990s. The first value was "people are basically good." He wrote that when eBay had only a few thousand users, because he believed it to be true. Now eBay has more than 200 million users, with more than a billion feedbacks a day, and the value is just as true now as it was then. eBay can be viewed as a giant social experiment, one that is dependent on human goodness to succeed. And the unprecedented success of eBay, around the world and in dozens of different cultures and languages, serves as an emphatic assurance of the truth of that first value.

It is crucial to my argument that not just face-to-face, but also large-scale social organizations (as in eBay's "giant social experiment") can run on the basis of the Golden Rule or, simply put, on trust and honesty. eBay is the classic global village, spread out over every continent, and yet it works. In fact, it works on the same principles as you would expect an actual village to work. This is because the *capacity* for trust is a constant in human nature. It is not contingent on whether people know each other or can identify some specific affiliation (e.g., the same town, school, or religion). While levels of trust will vary with the situation, our capacity to develop trust—fueled by natural empathy—is always present. I will come back to this persistence later, when I address recent arguments that question the biological basis of moral behavior. But for now, I want to emphasize that knowing that we are moral actors—as Omidyar clearly did when starting out with eBay—is useful, not just in organizing personal relations but also in building vast businesses. If Omidyar had not understood that we are naturally moral actors, he would not have had the insight to invent eBay, much less the courage to risk its success in the market.

In "Reflections on an Initial Trust-Building Model," McKnight and Chervany studied the trust levels prevalent in e-commerce, and came to a startling conclusion: they are actually improved by the parties' distance and the lack of prior relationship. That is, the parties' natural trust has no major obstacles, and so, when supported by reliable software, it simply governs: "Initial trust appears most applicable in what might be called 'distant relationships.' Perhaps one reason initial trust principles work for e-commerce . . . is because of the social distance between the players." This backs up Rule's observation of people's good behavior on eBay. In fact, Rule points out that more than 99% of eBay transactions work out successfully: "Yes, there are bad guys, and yes, people do mistreat each other on eBay from time to time. But it's always less than 1% of the overall volume, which is a staggeringly low amount, when you think about it." When a dispute does arise, eBay encourages the parties to "communicate" in an effort to reach a resolution. More than half of the disputes are resolved in this manner, without ever having to engage eBay's online dispute resolution system (which effectively allows information technology to make the decisions). Presumably, if the disputing parties were encouraged to apply the same principles that Omidyar did when he founded eBay, that proportion would be even higher.

As Nobel laureate Kenneth Arrow has observed, "Virtually every commercial transaction has within itself an element of trust." Trust is enhanced when ABT is understood.

WHAT ABOUT THE LAW ITSELF?

ABT, understood in a legal context, offers the possibility of a fundamental change in jurisprudence through the introduction of Golden

Rule thinking. In an article on law and neuroscience, we suggest that recent work in neuroscience pointing toward a physical/hormonal basis for moral reciprocity—the "do unto others" dictum commonly called the Golden Rule—may have implications for how legal concepts have developed and should be applied. We start from the assumption, however, that while neuroscience can now perhaps demonstrate that moral reciprocity is the product of how human brains have evolved, it would be facile to argue that the law simply reflects this evolution, and incorporates (or should incorporate) a "do unto others" ideology into its basic, jurisprudential structure. As Portia so cunningly proves in *The Merchant of Venice*, "the quality of mercy" is just one factor among many that is weighed by judges before they reach a legally acceptable decision.

In modern American jurisprudence, the Golden Rule has no place in a courtroom. Indeed, courts will routinely reverse a decision where one party was permitted to argue that members of a jury should put themselves in the plaintiff's place when deciding damages. In one important case, *Whitehead v. Kmart Corp.* (1998), the Fifth Circuit court rejected the linguistically archaic formulation of moral reciprocity—the "do unto others" dictum—so as to underscore how alien the notion is to a modern civil proceeding: "This court has forbidden plaintiff's counsel to explicitly request a jury to place themselves in the plaintiff's position and do unto him as they would have him do unto them." Thus while *Whitehead* acknowledges the phenomenon that we propose here, that is, that humans tend toward empathy, the case utterly banishes it as inimical to the formal administration of justice.

The ABT suggests that the court's position in *Whitehead* contravenes how we now understand the brain, that is, it flies in the face of how humans are wired. Consider the facts; In *Whitehead*, a woman and her teenage daughter sued a department store after two assailants abducted and robbed them in the store's parking lot. After the abduction, the assailants took turns sodomizing the woman outside her vehicle while the other held the daughter inside. At trial, plaintiff's counsel argued to the jury that:

> The incident took approximately two hours from when they were abducted to when they were released. And I calculated it, and that's 7200 seconds. And I want for you to just for a couple of seconds to see—when I say start, that's ten seconds. Ten seconds.
>
> And can you imagine how it would feel to have a knife in your side or a knife on your leg or a pistol on your neck for ten seconds?

In overruling the lower court, the Fifth Circuit held that "even assuming he was not explicitly invoking the Golden Rule, counsel was clearly inviting the members of the jury to put themselves in the place of the plaintiffs when deciding damages." The fact that the jury was asked to empathize—to do what juries often do without being encouraged—was grounds for reversal. It is as if, in putting a price on what those women endured, the jury was supposed to not even think about how they themselves might have felt during the ordeal.

What we think the law should consider is whether, given our current understanding of the brain, such wholesale dismissal of human empathy is still appropriate. Is there room for empathy in a courtroom dealing with issues that are usually left to actuaries? Should neuroscience be dismissed as "fuzzy" science when stacked up against hard financial calculation? At present, most courts would seem to say yes. In another damages case, *Alexander v. City of Jackson* (2008), this time involving the sexual harassment of firemen, a Mississippi district court relied on *Whitehead* to throw out a decision in which financial awards calculated down to the exact penny were found tainted by the jury's response to a Golden Rule argument.

What scares courts about relying on emotion in damages cases? As the court said in *Moody v. Ford Motor Co.* (2007), "A Golden Rule argument is 'universally recognized as improper, because it encourages the jury to depart from neutrality and to decide the case on the basis of personal interest and bias rather than evidence.'" The court set up a dichotomy—empathy on one side (bad) vs. neutrality/ rationality on the other (good)—and relied on the assumption that a Golden Rule argument improperly "encourages the jury to depart from neutrality and to decide the case on the basis of personal interest and bias rather than on the evidence." From a neuroscience perspective, it would have been interesting to ask jurors whether they felt comfortable being told that their feelings were out of bounds in this case, in which a young man was killed in a rollover accident, and his parents' counsel appealed to the jury's own sense of personal fragility:

> It's going to happen. It might happen when you're on your way to school. It might happen when your mom takes your kids to day care. It might happen when you're in a rush to work. It might happen because a child runs in front of you, and you try to avoid it, It's going to happen.

In the dock, isn't this nightmare what everyone was quietly confronting? How could they not have been? What we want to present is evidence that courts might at least consider when examining how juries are motivated and whether those motivations are fair to all parties.

According to the *Moody* court, empathic feelings have no place in awarding damages because comparing oneself to the victim is *ipso facto* unfair: "Plaintiff's counsel's remarks in this case went to the likelihood that jurors would suffer a personal injury similar to that suffered by plaintiff's decedent…, and he asked the jurors to award damages as if they had been personally harmed." Why should the law diverge so much from how people naturally react, especially because we now *know* that the brain pushes us in the direction of empathy? Is there something special about the law such that it *should* require us to forego empathy? The *Moody* court starts from an assumption, which is suspect from a neuroscience point of view, that reason and disinterest are corrupted by identification with another human being—at least insofar as we are called upon to award that person monetary damages: "Because of the prejudicial nature of these arguments and the likelihood that these statements aroused the passions of the jurors, plaintiffs' counsel's Golden Rule arguments should be considered as a factor in ruling on the fairness of the trial as a whole."

We take the position that normal people—the kind who normally get onto juries—naturally shrink from doing harm. In a legal context, where harm is ritualized and can include failure to adequately compensate someone for a wrong that he has suffered, we think it is *natural*—and potentially desirable—that jurors be permitted to at least register feelings of personal identification. An appropriate degree of leeway in this regard could mitigate harm that might otherwise be done through a failure to empathize. The neuroscience discussion in this chapter is meant to justify this recommendation, and to demonstrate that splitting legal processes off from natural human empathy may take too harsh a view of empathy. Empathy is not mere, uncontrolled passion, but rather an instinct for avoiding another's harm. Viewed in this context, is there harm in seeking to avoid harm?

In some connections, legal institutions already take account of our instinct to identify with others, and to trust that because we extend ourselves they will reciprocate. Every society since the Phoenicians has had some form of contract law, in which individuals undertake to satisfy each other's expectations. While the law has built up extensive mechanisms to compensate for non-performance, and in some cases to ensure that the parties operate in good faith, the fact is that no procedures for reciprocal exchange could operate in the absence of trust. Contract law is built on the assumption that I would *prefer* your performance to any form of compensation, and that you *understand* my preference sufficiently so as to endeavor to meet it. In the law, a contract is "the meeting of minds," not just intellectually but also in terms of a shared will to perform. This sharing is antecedent to any formal legal arrangement, and makes such arrangement plausible, indeed possible. In other words, the legal institution of contract is a constructive example of how mutual identification can operate constructively within a legal framework.

There is a substantial body of scholarship on the role of good faith in contract law—what it means, where it should be applied, whether it can be enforced. Our evidence suggests, however, that the very notion of contract, that is, of mutual reciprocal undertaking, could not have developed (and could not operate practically) unless people believed in the basic responsiveness of others. That responsiveness, we argue, emanates from a mutual identification among contractual partners sufficient so that each partner will be motivated to avoid harming the others. In practical terms, that means that if you hire me to perform some task, I will actually try to do it. Just like you, I will want to maintain my reputation in the community, and I will want to earn money rather than owe it. If legal institutions can take on board these basic notions, now reinforced by brain research, then perhaps this type of understanding is possible in other areas of the law.

Though I have just cited tort and contract law, where in one sense there is less at stake, I would also like to say a word about criminal law. If it is true that humans are naturally motivated to shrink from harming other people, then what are the implications for someone who, for example, has committed first degree murder, and deliberately undertaken egregious harm? Does neuroscience suggest that this person is somehow not wired like most of us, and that his "fault" is more anatomical than moral? Arguments about mental capability have been around for a long time in establishing *mens rea*, and courts continue to wrestle with the issues. We are uncertain as to how the research discussed here should affect criminal law, but we think it should be examined as the law moves forward.

We recognize that there is serious, principled opposition to any such enterprise. Stephen Morse, from the University of Pennsylvania, for example, argues that even such high-profile cases as *Roper v. Simmons* (2005), holding that "juvenile offenders cannot with reliability be classified among the worst offenders," do not constitute a green light. Rather, he notes that while "perhaps the neuroscience evidence [offered by numerous *amici*] actually played a role in the decision...there is no evidence in the opinion to support this speculation." In adolescents, he claims that "at most, the neuroscientific evidence provides a partial causal explanation of why the observed behavioral differences exist and thus some further evidence of the validity of the behavioral differences. It is only of limited and indirect relevance to responsibility assessment, which is based on behavioral criteria." In effect, Morse reads *Roper* as an implicit rejection of neuroscientific evidence for the purpose of determining *mens rea*, as the Court failed to explicitly rely on what amounted to copious legal arguments in favor of such evidence.

Morse is in fact highly skeptical with regard to using neuroscience evidence for purpose of establishing responsibility, setting the bar so high that we think only a shift in the *nature* of such evidence (which we modestly claim to offer here) would stand even a chance of his seriously shifting his ground:

> Even if there were a perfect correlation between brain states and the behavioral criteria for responsibility, the brain states would be nothing more than evidence of the behavioral states. Such a correlation is a fantasy based on present knowledge and probably always will be when we are considering complex

human actions. If the person meets the behavioral criteria for responsibility, the person should be held responsible, whatever the brain evidence may indicate, such as the presence of an abnormality. If the person does not meet the behavioral criteria, the person should be held not responsible, however normal the brain may look. Brains are not held responsible. Acting people are.

For Morse, neuroscientists demonstrate a reductive confusion concerning the relation between the brain and complex, intentional action. Our response is that at least so far, no one has raised the issue of empathy—that is, our apparently built-in capacity to resist doing harm—which we believe could constitute a game-changer insofar as how neuroscientific evidence might be of use in determining criminal responsibility. If in fact a court were not simply to confront a particular neuroscientific "state," but rather a fundamental failure to act on impulses basic to human nature, then perhaps the type of categorical opposition that Morse displays would not (at least immediately) be justifiable. We think such approach is worth a shot.

Indeed, in a more recent article, Morse conceded that neuroscience may *in the future* point the way toward "new or reformed legal doctrine," and may even contribute to the resolution of individual cases (albeit short of establishing *mens rea*). He makes this prediction based on the undeniable, rapid development of neuroscience, even though he cautions that it has not yet brought about any "paradigm shift in thinking about the nature of the person." However modestly, we think that ABT provides the instrumental evidence that Morse is hoping for.

We are encouraged by studies such as those of Henry T. Greely, who writes about the potential utility of neuroscience to the law. In a recent article, Greely provides a measured assessment of how neuroscience could affect the evaluation of *mens rea*:

> Neuroscience seems unlikely to lead to major changes in our view of criminal responsibility, but it will make a difference in some individual cases where it convinces us that the defendant truly and convincingly could not control his actions. Whether that means we treat him more leniently or more harshly is not clear, but we are likely, on occasion, to treat some defendants differently.

Like virtually all analysts, Greely is postulating that a complex calculus may develop whereby the acts of a particular individual, the circumstances of his action, and the potential of neuroscience to shed light on the underlying relevant motivations may yield guidance in criminal cases. We think that the virtue of our own approach—postulating an inborn proclivity toward empathy—is that it reinforces Greely's relative optimism toward the potential contributions of neuroscience by eliminating the need for ad hoc dependence on technology. If neuroscience can actually demonstrate that we are hard-wired for empathy, then virtually every case involving *mens rea* will, at some point and in some way, have to take account of why the defendant fell away from an empathetic norm. Thus whereas Greely suggests that on account of neuroscience evidence we may "on occasion... treat some defendants differently," we claim that we will always have to treat all defendants differently, taking into consideration a new array of variables.

What remains (apart from hoping that courts will acknowledge our position) is to work out what new tests should be introduced to make any departure from empathy (i.e., any apparent imbalance between prosocial and antisocial behaviors) an element in determining *mens rea*. Would this require relying on technology yet again? Possibly. But we think that establishing first principles must now be our first priority.

Of course, the law has its own conventions, and is not likely to change overnight. But as I mentioned previously, I think that the experience of eBay—now rivaled by a plethora of online auction sites, not to mention Amazon—lends support to an argument, based on ABT, that understanding how our brains are wired for empathy, and for basic decency toward one another, is useful knowledge, a meta-idea enabling us to organize society (even apart from the law) in ways that are more efficient and consistent with human nature. Yet as with disputes concerning the law, there are scholars who would claim just the opposite, and who argue that because we lie to each other all the time on the Internet the very notion of morality must be contingent, viable perhaps among small groups of near-affiliates but totally bankrupt in the world of postmodern theory, moral relativism, and virtual reality. The most cogent proponent of this idea is the eminent Harvard psychologist and MacArthur Fellow, Howard Gardner. In his recent book, *Truth, Beauty, and Goodness Reframed* (2011), Gardner defines "morality" as the sort of reciprocal benevolence that one encounters among members of small, tight-knit groups; he sees "ethics" as the more complex social relations that prevail in large groups where we each play multiple roles—for example, as citizens and workers—to get by. In the realm of "ethics" we are moral opportunists who define the Good in terms of what is good for us; the Golden Rule is a relic, applicable in Boy Scout troops and small towns. As a consequence, Gardner argues that we need to "reframe" goodness contextually, so that in our postmodern, relativistic world we inhabit our various roles honestly and with honor. He insists that because we must now devise new, workable values, many "important considerations undermine any attempt to reduce human morality—let alone ethics—to a strictly biological account."

Of course, Gardner makes a powerful case, because we have all experienced shoddy service, misleading online come-ons, and weasel-words in trumped up resumes. Indeed, Gardner's chapter on "Goodness" offers numerous studies that, he argues, demonstrate the breakdown of decent social relations especially among the young, who illegally download copyrighted songs or do whatever it takes to get ahead. The picture is dismaying. Yet it's necessary to respond to this vision, as science has a great deal to say that is contrary.

First, to argue that humans are wired to be kind does not reduce morality to "a strictly biological account." I do not know any scientist who makes such a claim, and it is a caricature to suggest that one would. Scientists know that genes can express themselves—or not—based on various exogenous factors, and that it is only within this total picture that the bases of behavior are determined. Indeed, this book suggests that our best tendencies are *tendencies*, which we can consciously draw on to improve our conduct. Thus there is much that Gardner and I would agree on—for example, teaching business ethics has never been more crucial. But we differ dramatically over how to characterize our current moral climate and how to address its lapses. As the eBay example demonstrates, it is entirely possible for people to trust each other online, and even to resolve disputes growing out of online transactions. To argue, as Gardner does, that the online world is a moral travesty is simply wrong. Of course there is misinformation on the Internet, but when has there not been misinformation? In the 18th century, Daniel Defoe had more than 70 pseudonyms, and famously wrote on both sides of hot-button issues while pretending that none of those blasts were his. The difference is that now we have far greater access to misinformation, so it can do more damage. Yet such access, and the attendant risk, does not affect people's capacity for moral behavior. That remains the same.

Indeed, in a recent *Wall Street Journal* article ("Internet On, Inhibitions Off: Why We Tell All"), Matt Ridley noted that the anonymity of the Internet allows us to be *more* honest, to the point that we spill out our hearts and say what we think irrespective of whose ox is gored. John Suler of Rider University calls this extreme honesty "the online disinhibition effect," where because we are not looking someone in the eye we feel free to be hyper-candid. The argument is consistent with what I have been arguing, namely, that a community's size and impersonality need not cause people to lose their ability to be straight with each other; according to Ridley and Suler, that ability is actually increased.

Second, as I discussed earlier, conflict resolution is an extremely viable means to settle controversies, even though the people involved are strangers, inhabiting roles that make them citizens of Gardner's postmodern dystopia. Indeed, running through conflict resolution in its many forms is the *constant* ability of people to empathize and trust each other. Because empathy and trust operate as constants, even in the impersonal environments that Gardner suggests exhibit bad faith, it is apparent that his analysis does not fully encompass how the world operates. We can certainly raise the levels of empathy and trust in any given situation, but that does not mean that as a species we lack the inclination toward empathy and trust except with regard to our neighbors and kin.

My point, if I have not already made it clearly, is that the size and complexity of a community do not determine people's capacity to act morally. Of course, different groups will require various and specific moral guidance. Doctors rely on medical ethicists; police departments have internal affairs units; and even the *New York Times* has a Public Editor to keep its writers within journalistic norms. But the existence of such distinct moral formations does not mean that, as a whole, humans have shed any of their native moral capacities. It does mean that we should design methods to bring these capacities more immediately and vigorously into play. This is an organizational question, as well as a question of trial-and-error to see what works best to achieve this result. It does not, however, require an effort to bring us back from moral desuetude. Quite the contrary, to understand the Benevolent Brain and seek to apply it should be a cause for optimism.

Yet it is clear that until the nuanced arguments of modern neuroscience are more generally understood, such optimism will not be widely shared. In a review of Simon Baron-Cohen's *Zero Degrees of Empathy: A New Theory of Human Cruelty*, Andrew Scull issued the following broadside, a more technically adorned version of Gardner's misgivings:

> Throughout *Zero Degrees of Empathy*, there are claims about an ability to peer into the brain, to see what is happening in various regions of the brain, to be able to make a connection, through the miracles of functional MRIs, between brain and behaviour. This is, let us be blunt, nonsense. Despite important advances in neuroscience, we are very far indeed from being able to connect even very simple human actions to the underlying structure and functioning of people's brains.

Zero Degrees of Empathy, though authored by an eminent Cambridge psychologist, contains much that can be easily caricatured. What, for example, does Baron-Cohen mean by his core concept of "empathy erosion," where certain circuits in the brain fail to light up under the scrutiny of an fMRI? Where is such "empathy" located in the brain, and how is it eroding? Yet all the same, in criticizing this and other aspects of Baron-Cohen's work, Scull jumps overboard, segueing from a modest and correct appreciation of the limitations of fMRIs to a panic-stricken disavowal of the idea that modern neuroscience is perpetrating a reductionist approach to explaining human mentality and behavior. In hundreds if not thousands of cases, neuroscientists have succeeded in showing the causal connections between the structure and function of the human brain and human actions. True, most of those actions are relatively simple: straightforward perceptual abilities or simple motor acts. But the factual bases of such connections are undeniable. ABT builds on them, and deduces from them the sort of rational implications that scientists make all the time. To deny the facts on which ABT is based would be intellectually perverse; to do so would additionally deny the practical benefits of knowing that the genesis of altruistic behavior resides naturally in the brain.

Certainly, ABT, which is based in neuroscience, may not be inherently obvious in the following sense. To some skeptics, no theory relying on brain mechanisms can explain altruism. Yet while Gardner is pessimistic concerning a biological approach to human relations, he provides no adequate countervailing evidence. Moreover, the ethical universal that has served our species across the globe for thousands of years still applies. In our forebrains, the neural circuitry that produces altruistic behavior operates—as it always has—irrespective of any discursive distortions produced by postmodernism. Most importantly, a person's good self-image applies to his behavior online as much as it does to his behavior toward a neighbor. In fact, Gardner cites a key formative fact: the individual's "sense of identity," especially in young individuals. The data discussed in this chapter, showing the effect of teaching an individual that he is good by virtue of his brain's natural function, may lay part of Gardner's anxiety to rest.

Though he may not be aware of it, Gardner may actually agree with me regarding basic principles. He believes it is useful to offer children presentations of "impressive and convincing 'live' role models of behaviors and reasons," including "dramatizing the consequences for those who honor the codes and those who transgress." Such examples of good or bad behavior can easily be extended into the postmodern digital domain. Gardner may even be pointing toward the psychological power of Golden Rule neuronal circuitry when he states that "our notions of goodness, in the individual moral sense, are far more entrenched than our conceptions of beauty." They are entrenched because they have *been* entrenched along an evolutionary timescale. Our notions of our own goodness, buttressed by knowledge of our moral brains' capacities, operate as psychological forces for continued good behavior both in our physical neighborhoods and in the digital world.

ABT demonstrates, even to people who are skeptical of others, that there is ground for hope, that is, hope that other people are not merely opportunists and egocentrics but rather available—like the rest of us—to engage in close friendships. Even for those people who have been harmed as youngsters, whether by parents, intimates, or perhaps abusive clergy, retraining in the nature of their own moral circuitry and that of others may help to reestablish the capacity for trust and friendship.

That ABT changes our perception of altruism itself is implicit in this chapter. Knowing that beneficent behavior is an inevitable, natural property of our neuronal circuitry lifts golden rule behavior out of the realm of religion and places it in the realm of natural science. It is a natural component of what makes us tick.

WRAPPING UP

In conclusion, if a person simply realizes that he is wired for good, altruistic behavior, and behaves accordingly, and if the person toward whom he is about to behave does the same thing, then everything is likely to come out OK. Of course, though such operations on oneself as decision maker are well and good, what about the social milieu in which the decision maker operates? The very last chapter will address this question as it discusses social applications of Altruistic Brain thinking.

FURTHER READING

C. D. Allis, ed. 2007. *Epigenetics*. Cold Spring Harbor, NY: Cold Spring Harbor Press.

D. Ariely. 2012. *The Honest Truth About Dishonesty: How We Lie to Everyone— Especially Ourselves*. New York: HarperCollins.

R. Bachmann and A. Zaheer, eds. 2006. *Handbook of Trust Research*, pp. 29–51. Cheltenham, UK: Edward Elgar.

L. Blackwell, K. Trzesniewski, and C. Dweck. 2007. "Implicit Theories of Intelligence Predict Achievement Across an Adolescent Transition: A Longitudinal Study and an Intervention." *Child Development* 78, 246–263.

R. Davidson and S. Begley. 2012. *The Emotional Life of Your Brain: How Its Unique Patterns Affect the Way You Think, Feel and Live—and How You Can Change Them*. New York: Hudson Street Press.

Howard Gardner. 2012. *Truth, Beauty and Goodness Reframed*. Cambridge, MA: Harvard University Press.

Mary Gordon and Daniel Siegel. 2009. *Roots of Empathy: Changing the World Child by Child*. New York: The Experiment LLC.

V. Job, C. Dweck, and G. Walton. 2010. "Ego Depletion—Is It All in Your Head? Implicit Theories about Willpower Affect Self-regulation." *Psychological Science* 21, 1686–1693.

Jerome Kagan. 1992. *Unstable Ideas: Temperament, Cognition, and Self*. Cambridge, MA: Harvard University Press.

Jerome Kagan. 2010. *The Temperamental Thread: How Genes, Culture, Time and Luck Make Us Who We Are*. New York: Dana Press.

Jerome Kagan and Nancy Snidman. 2009. *The Long Shadow of Temperament*. Cambridge, MA: Harvard University Press.

J. Mangels, B. Butterfield, J. Lamb, J., C. Good, and C. Dweck. 2006. "Why Do Beliefs about Intelligence Influence Learning Success? A Social Cognitive Neuroscience Model." *Social Cognitive and Affective Neuroscience* 1, 75–86.

Bruce McEwen. 2010. *Adverse Childhood Experiences*. New York: Dana Press.

C. McEwen and R. Maiman. 1984. "Mediation in Small Claims Court: Compliance Through Consent." *Law & Society Review* 18, 1–39.

C. McEwen, R. Maiman, and L. Mather. 1994. "Lawyers, Mediation, and the Management of Divorce Practice." *Law & Society Review* 28, 149–186.

D. Harrison McKnight and Norman L. Chervany. "Reflections on an Initial Trust-Building Model." https://www.msu.edu/~mcknig26/Reflections.pdf,

R. Pearce and R. E.Wald. 2011. "The Obligation of Lawyers to Heal Civic Culture: Confronting the Ordeal of Incivility in the Practice of Law." *University of Arkansas at Little Rock Law Review* 34; *U Denver Legal Studies Research Paper* No. 11–27; *Fordham Law Legal Studies Research Paper* No. 1969961. SSRN: http://ssrn.com/abstract=1969961

Donald Pfaff and Sandra Sherman. 2010. "Possible Legal Implications of Neural Mechanisms Underlying Ethical Behavior." In M. Freeman, ed., *Law and Neuroscience—Current Legal Issues*, Vol. 13, pp. 419–432. Oxford: Oxford University Press.

Elena Rocco. 1998. "Trust Breaks Down in Electronic Contexts but Can Be Repaired by Some Initial Face-to-Face Contact." In *Proceedings of the SIGCHI Conference on Human Factors in Computing Systems*. New York: ACM-Addison Wesley, pp. 496–502. http://social.cs.uiuc.edu/class/cs598kgk-04/papers/p496-rocco.pdf

Colin Rule. 2002. *Online Dispute Resolution for Business*. San Francisco: Jossey-Bass.

[7]

WHY THE ALTRUISTIC BRAIN MATTERS

Its Significance to Addressing Individuals' Bad Behavior

Altruistic Brain mechanisms are powerful, predisposing humans to act with reciprocal kindness. Nevertheless, other mechanisms built into the brain can challenge them, producing aggressive, antisocial behaviors that probably evolved to protect us against threats extant in early human history. As a neuroscience theorist, I must deal with these antisocial behaviors.

Of course, we may not need these protective behaviors anymore, at least to the same degree, as civilization (with its constraints and moral dicta) is itself our primary protection. But because the brain has not evolved at the pace of civilization (and because we are not always as civilized as we should be) we still must find ways to control antisocial tendencies that are part of our neuroanatomical/neuro-chemical inheritance. This chapter seeks to explain the physical bases of these tendencies so that we can begin to deal with them. Once we appreciate the relationship between Altruistic Brain mechanisms and those in our brains that give rise to baser impulses, we can create social conditions that give the Altruistic Brain wider scope in the face of our own natural pushback. In a book about our natural predisposition toward altruistic behavior, it would be ludicrous to ignore criminal and other egregious forms of behavior that we see all around us. Nor would I rationalize these behaviors, and suggest that they are less egregious than they seem. Rather, this chapter will argue that humans are equipped to regulate and limit these behaviors, provided that conditions encourage them to do so. A neuroscientific understanding of antisocial behaviors should help to deter them.

Thus though this chapter addresses aggression and sexual violence—behaviors not generally associated with our capacity to empathize—it is important to understand that the balance between our good and bad tendencies is not fixed; it can be altered toward the good. To think about how this might come about, we need to understand what makes us bad, as well as the interplay among various factors that tip the balance in one direction or the other.

In his recent book, *The Social Conquest of Earth,* the Harvard biologist Edward O. Wilson cites continuing battles in the human mind between selfish instincts and the forces of altruism. Sometimes altruism wins. Sometimes it doesn't. In cases such as the latter, the wiring for altruistic behavior has malfunctioned, or competing motives such as greed have overcome "forces for good." There are many reasons why this occurs, some of which are detailed here. The Altruistic Brain will or will not work depending on the strength of various neurochemical reactions, and this serves to provide the nexus between the science of reciprocity and the science of self-interested nastiness. Of course, while I offer an explanation of this nexus, it is clear that neurochemistry and a person's social/cultural environment work together to create—and regulate—behavior. Chapter 8 will discuss the effect of environment. But at this point, we first need to grasp the brain's role in originating bad behavior.

In E. O. Wilson's terms, when tendencies against empathic behavior "win out" over Altruistic Brain mechanisms, science usually can provide no specific—or rather, complete—explanation of how that occurs. In the cases discussed later, however, the hormonal or genetic influences on the nervous system are clear enough that a scientist can provide some insight. This is because the initial strength and reliability of Altruistic Brain mechanisms can vary widely from one individual to another. Our focus here is on the behaviors of individuals whose mechanisms are weak. For example, their image-merging operation (Step 3, as discussed in Chapter 2) may be deficient on account of a neurological quirk.

TESTOSTERONE-FUELED AGGRESSION; VIOLENT CRIME

Let's start by discussing male violence. Obviously, "violence" is not just male and not just physical. But I begin with male aggression because modern science has had its best success explaining this subject as compared to other forms of antisocial behavior. Male aggression is the paradigmatic form of bad behavior, enabling us to work toward understanding other forms. Beyond current data, I envision an array of antisocial behaviors—physical and mental, male and female—as part of a spectrum of challenges to the Altruistic Brain. Once we understand the basic neurochemistry underlying these behaviors, and begin to address their environmental counterparts, we can seek to create the countervailing circumstances that will minimize their effects on the Benevolent Brain.

While most violence is physical, it can also be psychological. However, physical violence is the kind of antisocial behavior most easily explained by 21st century neuroscience because it is most clearly linked to biological factors. Internationally, more than 85% of murders are committed by men. In the United States, men initiate more than 90% of violent acts. Young white males between 14 and 24 years of age, though only 6% of the US population, commit almost 17% of the murders; young black males in the same age range, only 1.2% of the population, account for 27%. Together, these two groups—just over 7% of the population—commit 45% of the homicides. As Steven Pinker observed in *The Better Angels of Our Nature,* "Though the exact ratios vary, in every society, it is the males more than the females who play-fight, bully, fight for real, rape, start wars and fight in wars." Chris Kojm, Chairman of the National Intelligence Council, has stated that in areas where there are disproportionate numbers of young men, the risk of genocide increases. Not unrelated, when James Holmes murdered 12 people in Aurora, CO in July, 2012, Erika Christakis, a public health advocate and Harvard College administrator, cited "the glaring reality that acts of mass murder (and, indeed, every single kind of violence) are overwhelmingly perpetrated by men."

Violence against women occurs with alarming frequency, and some murders committed by women result when they defend themselves against men. According to a United Nations General Assembly study, "at least one out of every three women around the world has been beaten, coerced into sex or otherwise abused in her lifetime, with the abuser typically someone she knows." But while women are frequently victimized, defenselessness in general seems to be a goad to violence.

Consider the common occurrence of a spurned male lover who stalks and violently attacks his ex-girlfriend. What neurochemical factors in the male brain are responsible for such violence? No surprises here; testosterone, having been produced by the testes and circulated in the bloodstream to the brain, promotes activity in neural circuits that will produce aggressive behavior and suppress activity in neural circuits that would reduce aggression. Both of these actions prime the trigger for violent behavior (see Figure 7.1). Lipid-soluble (that is, fat-soluble) testosterone spreads from the bloodstream through the entire brain, which has a great deal of lipid. In neurons, testosterone has two types of actions. First, a select group of neurons (called androgen receptors because testosterone is an androgenic hormone) contain proteins that are specialized to bind up testosterone (Figure 7.2). ("Androgenic" derives from the Latin *andro* ["male"] and *genic* ["making"]). As soon as

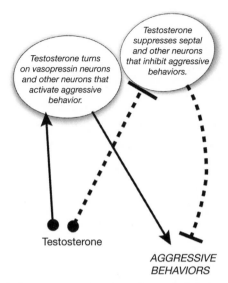

Figure 7.1 The hormone testosterone has at least two different ways of promoting impulsive physical aggression.

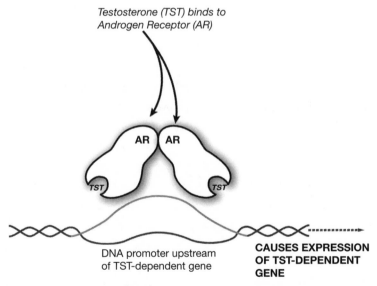

Figure 7.2 Testosterone (TST), a hormone that promote impulsive aggressive behavior, enters the nerve cell and, in the nerve cell nucleus, binds to a specific protein, the androgen receptor (AR). Then, after the AR binds to DNA, TST-dependent genes that affect aggressive behavior can be turned on.

testosterone has bound to its androgen receptor in a neuron, the receptor protein finds its way to the surface of the DNA in that neuron and has the opportunity to alter gene expression.

Most important for production of aggressive behavior by nerve cells in the forebrain is testosterone's stimulation of gene expression from the vasopressin gene, where "expression" means to make the gene's corresponding RNA, and thence the protein that contains the vasopressin. Vasopressin, in turn, can facilitate aggressive behavior by males. Smaller than the smallest proteins, vasopressin acts in certain parts of the midbrain, toward the top of the brainstem, to facilitate aggressive behaviors in laboratory animals. It acts the same way in humans. Intranasal administration of vasopressin has been reported to promote aggression in men. Blocking access to vasopressin receptors reduces aggressive behaviors. An ancient nine-amino-acid string evolved to yield, in mammals, oxytocin and vasopressin, oxytocin fostering friendly behaviors and vasopressin fostering aggressive behaviors.

Second, testosterone can also act rapidly at the membrane of a nerve cell and can alter the electrical activity of nerve cells. Exactly how such actions tie into aggressive behavior is not yet known, but it is easy to surmise that very rapid actions of testosterone in the brain could trigger impulsive acts of aggression.

Most of our knowledge about aggression mechanisms derives from animal research. This work has implications for humans. Consider eunuchs, for example, whose testes have been surgically removed. They have never been known to initiate physical aggression. At the other extreme, the overaggressive man is said to have "testosterone poisoning," so much testosterone circulating that his behavior is noticeably socially awkward.

Such testosterone-fueled aggression originates in ancient parts of our forebrain. One cell group, exquisitely sensitive to testosterone, promotes aggression, while the second cell group inhibits it.

Testosterone activates the former and inhibits the latter, thus foster-ing aggression through a dual "push/pull" set of mechanisms.

The simplest story of all in the human brain is the stimulation of men's physical violence by testosterone. Do the myriad studies of ani-mals that clearly demonstrate how the administration of testosterone leads to greater aggression also tell us something about male aggres-sion in humans? Yes. Harrison Pope of Harvard Medical School was the first to show that androgenic hormones such as testosterone prompted increases in behavioral aggression ranging from increased feelings of hostility to increased rates of homicide. And, as shown by Tom Hildebrandt of the Mount Sinai School of Medicine, we should really worry about the use of synthetic androgenic hormones (e.g., by adolescent boys who want to "bulk up") designed to work like testos-terone and to stay in the body for a long time. In the short term, these hormones can trigger "roid rage," embarrassing, disruptive, and even criminal behaviors. The long-term consequences of synthetic andro-genic hormone use are still unknown.

Testosterone-fueled aggression feeds into the formation of social roles, shown originally in animals, but applicable to humans as well. For example, in social hierarchies involved with sexual behaviors in nonhuman primates, Barbara Smuts, professor of anthropology at the University of Michigan, has studied primate species in which males are aggressive against females. Such behavior often occurs in context with sex, for example, against females that have refused to mate, or to minimize contact between females from the male's own group with males from another group.

Outside the sexual context, males may fight females during feeding competitions, in defense of a close female associate or her offspring, or even to punish a female for previous aggression. In retaliation, females may join forces to form coalitions against males, especially against strange males, protection of an adult female who has been attacked by a male, and, probably the most common situation, protection of infants. In addition to testosterone's effects on aggression, in humans testosterone also drives an entire repertoire of behaviors: staring, speech duration, bodily postures that display supremacy, and so forth, that can be interpreted as seeking to raise social status or dominance. Testosterone heightens responses to angry facial expressions, including elevated vigilance and elevated heart rate. Correspondingly, testosterone can reduce friendly relations with those whom the testosterone-laden individual expects to compete. In fact, in laboratory studies of peoples' reactions to faces, testosterone significantly reduced interpersonal trust, in that testosterone-treated subjects had a much harder time rating a person's picture "trustworthy." Based on animal studies, these testosterone effects will not just occur instantly, but instead will have started before and during adolescence.

Some of these effects on behavior may be characterized by a vicious circle. While testosterone heightens aggressive behavior, winning a fight can increase testosterone as well as sensitivity to testosterone in the brain, such that each effect multiplies the other. When a rhesus monkey wins a fight, testosterone levels in the blood go up. Following a win, the proteins that bind testosterone, androgen receptors, are present in higher levels in a part of the brain, the ancient forebrain, that regulates social aggression. Thus the more testosterone that is present, the greater the brain's sensitivity to testosterone. Testosterone leads to fighting, and winning leads to testosterone effects in the brain.

There is no doubt, therefore, that aggressive, violent behavior by men can be fueled by testosterone circulating in their blood and entering their brains. And perhaps some of the "normal" ambitions and initiatives owe some of their psychic energy to testosterone. At the other end of the spectrum covering normal and abnormal social behaviors, however, psychopathology is at the other extreme.

We can consider three ways to reduce boys' aggression. First, engaging boys in prosocial group activities before testosterone levels rise during adolescence will head off testosterone-laden trouble. Second, for boys who are already "off the deep end" with violent behavior, blocking the testosterone/vasopressin connection should help. Finally, modern behavioral neuroscience recognizes, in published work, that any pharmaceutical approach has to be accompanied by cognitive behavioral therapy.

PSYCHOPATHOLOGY

Unfortunately, there are people who can perform multiple antisocial acts with no sense of remorse. Altruistic Brain Theory (ABT) simply does not work in these people. Some of these are psychopaths, and the most famous among them populate the media. A psychopath engages repeatedly in antisocial behaviors that seriously hurt others and that are accompanied by passive indifference to the destructive consequences of his actions.

At the age of 81, the psychopath Whitey Bulger finally got caught after years on the run. He was subsequently convicted of 11 cold-blooded killings and a string of gangland crimes. In his youth, and then as a career criminal, he sprayed bullets around Boston during a criminal career of violence and corruption much ballyhooed in the popular press. A vicious psychopath, Bulger belongs to that 1% of the population that—right from the start—appears to have no moral compass of any sort.

James David Martin, another example of this group, was also recently caught. When he was 17 he murdered another boy (and stole his Air Jordan sneakers as well); went to jail; later stabbed another boy seriously after getting out of jail, having looped the drawstring of his sweatpants around the victim's neck; went to jail again; and then strangled his wife. Martin's "career" started early, as it does in many cases. As an eight-year-old boy he cut up trousers with a scissors and pulled all his hair out. Beyond Martin, it is easy, unfortunately, to cite other examples. For instance, another young psychopath killed the family cat. A third child pushed a toddler into the deep end of a swimming pool and calmly watched him drown. As reported by Jennifer Kahn, these children had no remorse or empathy, and have been labeled "callous-unemotional." Indeed, in an analysis of Eric Harris, one of the teenage murderers in the Columbine massacre, Dave Cullen remarks that "Mr. Harris kept a sort of journal for an entire year, focused largely on his plan to blow up his school and mow down survivors with high-powered rifles.... It's hate-hate-hate all the way through. He was a cold-blooded psychopath, in the clinical use of that term. He had no empathy, no regard for human suffering or even human life." These children and teenagers have already crossed the line into psychopathic behavior. Psychopathic adults were seriously antisocial children, and if the trouble starts so early then something must be seriously able to interfere with "Golden Rule wiring." Moreover, the genes determining sex do matter in this regard. According to British psychologist Sir Michael Rutter, psychopathological disorders that begin early in life feature a male predominance, while those with adult-onset emotional disorders a more frequently female one.

A psychopath can hurt others in many ways, not limited to the testosterone-fueled violent behavior that I just cited. A psychopath's predatory behavior, causing pain or loss to others, comes from a callous individual who acts without remorse. For reasons that Simon Baron-Cohen, professor of psychology at the University of Cambridge, has begun to address, the psychopath lacks empathy and the ability to be aroused by concern for someone who suffers from his criminal acts. As opposed to criminals who act for money, psychopaths, in the words of University of Virginia professor Jon Haidt, have "greater willingness to violate moral concerns of any type." Indeed, some men, by sudden, unpredictable outbursts terrorize those in their social and professional environments. They reach a level of psychological violence that, though not producing direct physical harm, has consequences that may be just as severe.

Baron-Cohen seeks to understand antisocial behavior by characterizing empathy according to degrees. People with a total absence of empathy ("Zero"), stuck in an environment with negative effects on their personalities ("Negative"), may well turn out to be psychopaths ("Zero-Negative Type P"). According to Baron-Cohen, the psychopath, totally preoccupied with his desires and willing to do whatever it might take to satisfy them, may be superficially charming, but will be undependable, dishonest, suffer from a poverty of emotions, and will fail to learn from punishment. Baron-Cohen traces the psychopath's life back to a condition of "insecure attachment" to his parents. To understand this, think about how the attachment theorist John Bowlby, referred to in Chapter 4, emphasized the infant's caregiver as a "secure base" to whom the infant, having begun to explore the world, can return for "emotional refueling." Baron-Cohen thinks that the psychopath-to-be lacks this resource. Such a person does not fear punishment for immoral acts, and so the barrier to committing immoral acts has been lowered. Aside from inadequate early support from parents or other caregivers, how did this come about?

Simple genetic determinism can be ruled out. No one has reported a "psychopath gene." Instead, experts have emphasized the importance of genetic influences interacting with environmental influences. For example, mutations in genes connected with signaling by the neurotransmitter serotonin *coupled with* a crime-ridden environment might predetermine the kind of impulsive aggressive behavior sometimes associated with psychopathology. This is important because we can deal with environmental influences, and attempt to compensate for them so as to rectify the lack of empathy. Also, these new theories lead us to take an activist role, promoting conditions that allow the Altruistic Brain to operate unimpeded by negative influences. In other words, understanding what can go wrong with "golden rule" brain wiring does not just give us more science. Rather, it allows us to consider how—by addressing the interaction of such wiring with a person's environment—we can make the world better one person at a time. It does no good only to understand how *either* the brain *or* the environment conduces to psychopathic behavior; it is crucial to fully understand both so that we can take a holistic, scientific, and cultural approach to addressing a person's psychopathology.

Indeed, current neuroscience evidence demonstrates that the combination of genetic and environmental events must affect brain circuits to permit the emergence of psychopathologic behavior. A large number of studies of cerebral activity in psychopaths compared it to activity in the brains of control subjects. Several different brain imaging techniques were used. It was common to find reduced activity in the prefrontal cortex of psychopathic subjects, which was significant because normal activity in the prefrontal cortex is required to support typical, civilized decision making, and in particular to suppress the output (including violent emotional behaviors) from the ancient forebrain underneath. In another study, highly aggressive people displayed less activity in a part of the prefrontal cortex especially devoted to emotional decision making, affecting the individual's choice of expressing one emotion rather than another. In another study, the higher a subject scored on a test of psychopathic personality traits, the less activity he had in this prefrontal brain region. Once one important area of the brain like the prefrontal cortex is knocked out of its normal mode of functioning, this may indicate that large-scale brain networks may be dysfunctional. Most important for the Altruistic Brain is that reduced prefrontal cortical activity would reduce the ability of the psychopathic brain to inhibit antisocial behavior.

If we could understand the neuronal or hormonal basis of psychopathology, we could predict it, prevent it, or both. Indeed, neuroscience has made strides in this direction. One doctor compared brain scans of eight psychopaths, as defined previously, with those of eight criminals who were not considered psychopaths, while they were required to rehearse and recognize a series of words. Some of the words—for example, "devastated," "death," or "cancer"—had the effect of inducing negative emotions, while others were emotionally neutral. Scientists already knew that normal volunteers would have a greater degree of activation in the ancient parts of the forebrain when performing this task with emotionally loaded words as opposed to neutral words. Psychopaths had significantly less activation in response to the emotionally loaded words than did criminal non-psychopaths, and this difference was seen only in parts of the forebrain connected with emotional responses: the amygdala, the cingulate cortex, and part of the frontal cortex. It is as though the psychopathic brain does not register an emotional reaction to things that a normal brain would react to strongly.

Kevin Dutton, professor at Magdalen College, Oxford, has a different take on psychopathology. He addresses some personal qualities of psychopaths, which he labels "grandiose sense of self-worth, persuasiveness, superficial charm, ruthlessness, lack of remorse and the manipulation of others." Then, surprisingly, he identifies these aspects of personality as frequent "hallmarks of success!" The cool neurosurgeon who, in the operating theatre, "cannot afford the luxury" of compassion for the patient he is operating on. The politician, running for high office, similarly, needs that superficial charm and capacity for manipulating others. In Dutton's view, these are the types of individuals who are actually making appropriate use of their "psychopathic" traits. In psychopaths, E. O. Wilson's "war" between good and bad impulses is over before it has even begun. Tendencies toward evil behavior, permitted by mechanisms that we still don't fully understand, overwhelm the neural circuitries that make up the Benevolent Brain.

CORRUPTION

Up until now, this chapter has discussed hormonal and genetically based tendencies that can overwhelm the Altruistic Brain, leading to antisocial behavior Now, however, I want to discuss something much trickier: corruption, where the Altruistic Brain *itself* produces socially unacceptable acts. That is, in cases of corruption, the trigger mechanism in Step 5 is co-opted, turned back on itself so that though a type of reciprocity occurs it clashes with social norms. Brain mechanisms that normally function to produce "good," benevolent behavior result in behavior that society deplores. It is business-as-usual for the brain, an empathic burst where someone helps someone else; what makes corruption "bad" is the social mores that have grown up around it. Such mores demonize bribes and similar behavior that the brain recognizes as useful reciprocity. Put starkly, where the brain sees an opportunity to reciprocate—and hence foster mutual survival—the law sees illegality. Corruption is in this sense the limit case of ABT, at once proving its vitality even as it shows how in certain instances society will actually reject natural impulses toward mutual support that contravene norms that possess competing utility. We dislike corruption because it is seen to be unfair to society *at large*; as between the parties engaged in corruption, however, it's just fine. Thus though no respectable scientist could ever justify corruption, I think it's important to demonstrate its uncanny affiliation to some of our best instincts.

Some people think of corruption as a set of cold, calculating acts by public figures or public organizations, acts carried out in a brutal fashion. But by far the largest numbers of corrupt acts, numerous because they are so easy, occur among friends and acquaintances on a small, local scale: the policeman in a tough neighborhood who gets free food at the deli and who, in turn, promises to fix the deli owner's parking tickets; the financier who provides inside information to the broker who gives him a price break; the building inspector who overlooks a violation so that his nephew can rent space on the cheap. Here is a classic case: Rajat Gupta, the retired head of McKinsey and former Goldman Sachs board member, was convicted in July, 2012, of conspiracy and securities fraud for leaking boardroom secrets to the billionaire hedge fund manager Raj Rajaratnam (himself convicted of insider trading). In pronouncing on the case, the prosecutor observed that "Rajaratnam offered Gupta many benefits. What was good for Rajaratnam and Galleon [the fund that he managed] was good for Gupta." That is, though each benefited the other, their actions were illegal.

Of course, millions of corrupt acts occur every year, even if most are too petty to be prosecuted. In the stepped illustration that follows, I demonstrate how the deli owner, bribing the policeman, sets off the five neuronal "steps" involved with the Altruistic Brain, such that the policeman agrees to scrub the deli owner's tickets. The steps are exactly the same as if the policeman had discovered the deli owner slipping on the ice; the only difference is that in the case of corruption, the outcome is socially unacceptable.

How Corruption Works: An Illustration Using ABT

Deli Owner (D. O.)	Policeman (P)
Step 1. Envisions act (giving free donuts and coffee to policeman, P.).	1. Envisions act (to overlook parking violations).
Step 2. Perceives policeman, P.	2. Perceives deli owner, D. O.
Step 3. Merges images (P. with D. O.).	3. Merges images (D. O. with P.).
Step 4. Evaluates (yes, "nice" for D. O. and P.).	4. Evaluates (yes, "nice" for P. and D. O.).
Step 5. Decision. Gives free donuts and coffee to P.	5. Overlooks parking violations.

Criminology provides endless examples of corruption. Indeed, corruption has been cropping up forever and occurs worldwide. Its ubiquity fits perfectly with the Altruistic Brain, as our Golden Rule wiring is so reliable. Think of crony capitalism or (in its mob-inspired knock-off) the Mafia's "omerta" (its infamous code of loyalty and non-cooperation with authorities). Corruption is honor among thieves, and what in police circles is the Blue Wall of Silence, that is, no cop turns in another even if that results in obstruction of justice. (On June 25, 2012, the *New York Times* reported that an NYPD member who "ratted" on his peers said that he had been "banished to an island all by myself"). The scientific mechanisms for corruption are as clearly understood as for Golden Rule wiring *because they are the same*. It's just that corruption is illegal.

In the political sphere it occurs when government officials use their power for illegitimate private gain. Everyone remembers Illinois governor Rod Blagojevich, who—given his appointment power—tried to sell President Obama's vacated Senate seat to the highest bidder. "Blago" was part of a rich tradition of corruption in Illinois, where since the 1970s four out of seven governors have been convicted of it. In Chicago, dozens of aldermen and other officials have been similarly convicted. They have taken bribes, traded on their influence, extorted funds, and otherwise enriched themselves by abusing their office. It is precisely such trading—you scratch my back, I'll scratch yours—that brings corruption within the ambit of the Altruistic Brain.

But though Chicago was recently found to be the most corrupt city in America, it has no monopoly on such abuse. Construction site inspectors in New York City took bribes to cover up noncompliance. City laws for the safety of huge construction cranes were not followed. Even at Yankee Stadium, the cement was not inspected properly, nor, as it turns out, was a lot of other cement used in projects around town. On April 27, 2012, the *New York Times* carried a story about a convicted state senator from Brooklyn who, the judge said, had plunged "daggers in the heart of honest government" by taking hundreds of thousands of dollars in bribes to influence legislation. The brain's neurochemistry does not make distinctions between legal and illegal; rather, it sees the opportunity for reciprocity.

In the District of Columbia, Council members running unopposed still raked in fortunes by way of campaign contributions, and then showered their backers with tax preferences. Elsewhere in the District, disgraced Senator John Ensign was found by the Senate Ethics Committee to be seriously suspect when he pressured Nevada cronies to assign huge lobbying contracts to Douglas Hampton, a former aide. Ensign had been having an affair with Hampton's wife and, as the *Times* gamely observed, the deal was a means of "finding income for the aggrieved [Hampton] and containing the damage from the affair." Not mincing words, the ethics investigation found that Ensign had "used his office and staff to intimidate and cajole constituents into hiring Mr. Hampton." Ensign even continued his lobbying contacts with Hampton after having been warned of their likely illegality. Of course, the case provides a stark example of how the brain's processes diverge from those of society's, in this instance articulated by the Ethics Committee. Ensign offers Hampton something that Hampton needs—cash—and Hampton reciprocates with what Ensign needs: silence. That the plan went awry and was exposed was just an unintended (though in Washington, highly foreseeable) consequence.

Even rural America is not immune. In July, 2012, the *New York Times* ran an op-ed by Jason Howard, who has studied corruption in Appalachia. Howard observed that "After finally recognizing the union, [the big coal companies] opposed its demands for things like a living wage, health insurance, safety precautions and measures to curb the alarming rates of black lung disease. The strategy was simple: the companies would buy off individual communities and leaders, exchanging meager payouts for silence or even support against the more adamant activists." Appalachian communities are tight-knit, inbred places. Company execs might see some local "leader" in church or at a bar. Cutting a deal would be easy, especially since even the leaders were often working men with families to support and little to show for their work.

But lest we wring our hands over local politics and proverbial smoke-filled rooms, we should recognize that corruption knows no borders. This is because the brain knows no borders! In Africa, corruption has been a way of life. Congo's Mobutu Sese Seko secreted billions in bribes and pay-offs overseas. So did the generals running Nigeria. On June 11, 2012, the US Department of Justice charged Teodorin Obiang, the son of Equatorial Guinea's dictator, with taking massive bribes from foreign timber companies (often in cash-filled suitcases) which he laundered and spent in the United States. Obiang was Guinea's Forestry Minister, and was literally profiteering off the country's resources. Indeed, food and humanitarian aid in places like Somalia have routinely been stolen and sold by politicians while the people starve. As the great economist Amartya Sen has observed, food shortages are almost always a political phenomenon. Were Sen a neuroscientist, he would see the "politics" that he deplores in terms of a perverted moral reciprocity among corrupt leaders.

Under Vladimir Putin, Russia is awash in corruption: the country ranks 154th out of 178 in the Corruption Perception Index published by Transparency International. In a 2010 poll, 15% of Russians reported having paid a bribe. In China, people have died on account of corruption. Local officials, for example, allowed schools to be built that would collapse during an earthquake. The *Times* reported on April 26, 2012 that a Chinese government official steered business to Morgan Stanley in exchange for real estate secretly acquired on his behalf by a Morgan Stanley employee. In India, there were headlines over a hunger-striker willing to starve to death to call attention to official corruption.

Corruption, a "bad behavior" appropriate to this chapter, shows a modulation of the Altruistic Brain operation that we view in a darker hue. The mechanism is neutral; the interpretation defines the behavior as bad. Think about it. "You scratch my back and I'll scratch yours." Corrupt person A does a favor for person B, under the table, knowing that corrupt person B will, under the table, give something back. The examples given above could be multiplied by a thousand. Society makes distinctions that the brain does not. In each case, however, there is a perverse type of camaraderie that one can actually hear in the speech of corruption's participants. In the 2012 Barclay's Bank scandal, one trader emailed a colleague, "Dude, I owe you big time!...I'm opening a bottle of Bollinger," when the colleague had manipulated a rate and improved the trader's apparent profit.

OUR REACTIONS TO IMMORAL BEHAVIOR

The "disgust" reaction implicates how the Altruistic Brain functions. We learn from disgust, so that in the future we resist bad behavior when tempted. I will discuss how this reaction works, so that we can make the most of it in promoting prosocial behavior.

By "disgust," I mean the deeply negative impact that bad behavior produces on those who view such behavior but are not themselves affected by it (except, of course, to feel disgusted). Paul Rozin, professor of psychology at the University of Pennsylvania, has raised the possibility that the science of "gustation," that is, of taste, actually sheds light on the neuroanatomical pathways that mediate our innate, negative responses to immoral—that is, disgusting—behavior. He asks: Is moral disgust an elaboration of a food rejection system?" Certain bitter tastes and a whole variety of foods cause us to shrink away. Facial expressions and uncomplimentary words tell all nearby who see and hear that we don't want anything to do with that food. By implication, could the same neuronal system be involved with rejecting bad behavior?

Rozin raised the possibility that the very same neuronal systems that evolved to protect us from spoiled food also have been harnessed, during evolution of the brain (and of social life) to register our reactions to "disgusting" behaviors. According to that idea, we would react to witnessing obviously immoral behavior using the same neurons in the forebrain as we use to recognize disgusting tastes. As predicted by his early thinking, both muscular evidence and neuroanatomical evidence have supplied mechanisms and routes that link responses to disgusting tastes with responses to disgusting behaviors. At the muscular level, researchers at the University of Toronto recorded electrical signals from the muscles of the subjects' faces to compare reactions to disgusting foods and photographs with obviously unfair treatment at a "setup" economic game in the laboratory. One tell-tale muscle that raises the upper lip and wrinkles the nose was activated by bitter tastes and by photographs of things like feces. This same muscle was activated by the type of experimentally induced unfairness in a laboratory economic game that was so bad that the subject's response was characterized by a large degree of disgust. So, for this tell-tale facial muscle, there was equivalence. But how would the central nervous system react?

The best evidence for nervous system equivalence between terrible tastes and terrible behavior comes from a part of our cerebral cortex hidden from view, the insula (Figure 7.3). Long identified as a region of the cortex sensitive to signals from our viscera, our insular cortex can be visualized only if our temporal cortex has been "cut through," in a three-dimensional picture, and "flipped to the side." Neuroanatomists report that compared to other areas of our brains, the insula is "disproportionately enlarged" compared to monkey brains. These observations suggest that our brains correspondingly have a disproportionately large number of nerve cells devoted to increasing sensitivity to the moral quality of social acts. Most important, nerve cells there respond to tastes as well as to signals from our stomachs, bladders, and rectums. When volunteers were being brain-scanned while witnessing disgusting things or while they tasted

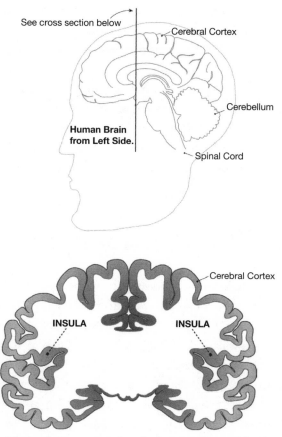

Figure 7.3 The insula is a region of cerebral cortex that is tucked beneath the cortical regions that you can usually see from the outside. Neurons in the insula may play a special role in avoiding immoral behavior that is "disgusting." Because older research had linked the insula to the sensory registration of "disgusting" tastes, Paul Rozin at the University of Pennsylvania came up with the phrase "from oral to moral."

bitter, disgusting liquids, their insula "lighted up." Further, when the insula is damaged, the experience of disgust is reduced. All of these observations support the "oral to moral" idea proposed by Paul Rozin, that the same brain region that responds to disgusting tastes also can be related to disgusting psychological situations, including morally disgusting acts. Moreover, because the function of disgust is to ensure avoidance of the object of disgust, it seems likely that even as we avoid eating garbage, we avoid distasteful social behavior.

So in the case of disgusting behavior and the insula, modern neuroscience has led us to an understanding about exactly where things can go haywire in the brain, resulting in unnatural antisocial or immoral behaviors. Of course, because some people do not always avoid distasteful behavior, the Altruistic Brain will on those occasions need strengthening. How can neuroscience suggest ways to prevent antisocial behavior?

STRENGTHENING THE ALTRUISTIC BRAIN

We have already seen how good social behavior is produced by brain "mechanisms" that constitute the Altruistic Brain. "Mechanisms" denote mechanical operations characteristic of a machine and, as we all know, any machine can fall apart. So while I have described how the mechanisms for moral instincts and ethical behavior work in the brain, I must accept that under some circumstances they simply will not work. Altruistic Brain circuitry can potentially be overwhelmed, particularly in crime-ridden environments. That is, even though Altruistic Brain circuitry is built into the human brain, we are also always subject to environmental influences. Someday completely different and interacting sets of pathologies—genetic, neuronal, environmental—might be seen to account for psychopathology. In any case, corruption, an anomalous outcrop of the ABT, uses Altruistic Brain circuitry albeit in ways that produce illegal results.

Potentially, Altruistic Brain mechanisms can be strengthened and, hence, their failure rate may be reduced. First, if possible, where young people are thought to be at risk of succumbing to antisocial instincts they should be supported and strengthened at the earliest opportunity. I am thinking of runaways; veterans who can't find work; as well as youngsters in halfway houses, juvenile detention centers, and the ones who bounce around in foster care until they "age out" and become homeless. In this population, we could, for example, measure the level of testosterone in a young boy's blood and saliva to see if it is off the charts. In not too long, scientists will be able to identify genetic sequences that predispose individuals toward antisocial behavior. The point is that we have the tools, and are acquiring more so that timely, humane intervention is possible, permitting natural human tendencies to prevail against countervailing natural predispositions.

Second, the environment that people inhabit should be optimized for good behavior. In the case of young people, we should examine the environments that parents provide—are the parents drug addicts, or just working so hard that they are never around? Where people are older, we should examine the psychological effects of run-down, ugly neighborhoods—the so-called "broken window" theory that repulsive surroundings lead to repulsive behavior. Schools and local institutions can foster self-esteem, as can simply having a job. Where people feel that they "belong," they will resist the pull of gangs, crime, and self-destructive relationships.

Third, when someone has exhibited antisocial behavior, measures must be taken to prevent its recurrence. Behavioral modification techniques and medical approaches have to be improved. As we have already seen, efforts to teach empathy are encouraging, and can be made even better by allowing individuals to understand that their brains incline toward empathy. ABT is not just the result of neuroanatomical analysis; it is instrumental, so that along with other instrumentalities in society it can be deployed to help bring antisocial individuals into the mainstream.

I am particularly encouraged by the work of neuroscientists who are studying the brain's plasticity, its ability to change *structurally* in response to experience, particularly such experience as is associated with mental effort. In this regard, what if we could increase the performance of the brain's neuronal circuitry (i.e., its neuronal structure) responsible for good behavior? This type of speculation is not far-fetched, and has already been vindicated in context with the practice of some forms of meditation. At the Laboratory for Affective Neuroscience at the University of Wisconsin, researchers working with psychology professor Richard Davidson found that continued Buddhist meditation *could* change structures in the brain. Likewise, Dr. Daniel Siegel, Director of the Mindful Awareness Research Center at UCLA, observes that "we can use [the developing ability to focus on our inner world] to resculpt our neural pathways, stimulating the growth of areas that are critical to mental health." If we can accomplish this resculpting and improve our mental health, could it also possible to do so with regard to the state of our morality?

Davidson actually comes closest to answering this question in the positive, in that his recent results affirm that our brains are dynamic organs, which can change over time in response to experience. He argues that we can exercise our brains, as we might our biceps or even our heart, and create new neural patterns that favor new behaviors. If biceps get stronger when we lift 50- and then 60-pound weights, likewise the brain can respond when we "practice" being good. It puts down neural patterns that make such behavior more and more automatic. Davidson suggests that good behavior is thus a skill and, like physical exercise, it gets easier as we keep at it. That is, the brain adapts, establishing neural pathways that accustom us to continued good behavior. In his most recent book, *The Emotional Life of Your Brain*, he observes that "[N]ature has endowed the human brain with a malleability and flexibility that lets it adapt to the demands of the world it finds itself in. The brain is neither immutable nor static but continuously remodeled by the lives we lead."

Such adaptations could be straightforward: laying down new synaptic connections. Or they could be more subtle: so-called "epigenetic" changes in which long-term alterations in the control of gene expression in certain neurons alter the performance of the Altruistic Brain circuitry. So if we already *possess* such circuitry, then we must be encouraged to use to use it on a regular basis. Our brains— our neural circuitry—should respond to this encouragement.

Moreover, if we *understand* that we already possess such circuitry, then the job becomes that much easier—who doesn't want to go with the flow? The point is to be continually encouraged, especially at a young age. Parenting experts, for example, will want to design methods that reinforce children's best instincts. Much work has been done on habit formation (why we bite our nails or turn the TV on before breakfast); this same line of research could turn toward how we get in the habit of being kind. Once we do get into the habit, the brain's adaptation will make that habit a more consistent part of our nature.

Despite our Altruistic Brain mechanism—and even our potential understanding of it—some people will give in to temptation, especially where they act intuitively or impulsively. Consider Bernard Madoff, who allowed himself to make quick bets that failed, and then allowed his errors to compound instead of admitting them. Madoff's flawed responses lead directly to this chapter's next section.

APPLICATION OF ABT IN BUSINESS AND OTHER SOCIAL ENVIRONMENTS: SLOWING DECISIONS TO AVOID SNAP JUDGMENTS AND IMPULSIVE BEHAVIOR

Neuroscientists and their natural partners, behavioral scientists, have led us to an understanding of two systems in the brain that regulate behavior over two entirely different time courses.

Consider good decisions and good behavior and the tempo at which they occur. Even though Altruistic Brain operations can operate rapidly and unconsciously to produce empathic behavior, they do not correspond to mere impulsiveness. On the average, well-considered, thoughtful approaches to ethical decisions will produce better, more prosocial behavior than thoughtless, impulsive approaches. In business, for example, when men have allowed their mistakes to multiply and get out of control, they may tumble (if only out of desperation) into terrible ethical lapses.

Now for bad behavior. How do we explain deviations by individuals from the kind of behavior that Altruistic Brain wiring predicts? Let's return to the financial outlaw, Bernard Madoff, and examine his acts more closely from a particularly neuroscience perspective. In *The Wizard of Lies*, Diana Henriques provides no real explanation of what motivated Madoff's behavior, despite offering masses of detail concerning his financial maneuvers. We read about his being caught up in the over-the-counter stock market in his early days and, subsequently, his feelings of obligation to erase losses that his early mistakes caused; this began the explosion of deceitful practices that over decades resulted in billions of dollars of loss. But there is no personal insight into his psychopathology. Coverage of Alan Sanford, the Texas fraud, displayed similar problems. We know that though both men began with reckless, thoughtless behavior, they got in much deeper than they intended...but what were they thinking along the way? More to the point, *how* were they thinking? Some recent work on how we *should* think sheds light on this question.

In *Blind Spots*, Max Bazerman and Ann Tenbrunsel focus on *unintentional* ethical lapses. Consider the explosion of our space shuttle *Challenger*, the result of the contractor company Morton Thiokol's ignoring its own engineer's warning about launching at low temperature, a mistake demonstrated later in a public hearing by the Nobel laureate physicist Richard Feynman. Consider as well the oil rig disaster in the Gulf of Mexico, caused by BP's determination to finish the rig's assembly, cut costs, and begin production. In *so many* cases, Bazerman and Tenbrunsel write, our "should brain" is over-come by our "want brain," which governs how people actually make decisions having moral import rather than how people would make such decisions in some ideal world. Rapid, impulsive, selfish instincts win out over slower, prosocial mental processes. We might say that a psychopath lacks moral awareness or moral intention and thus does not act in a moral fashion, but as scholars in the new, empirical field of Behavioral Ethics, these authors want to know what that phrase means in terms of brain function and behavior.

Two groups of scholars from interesting but disparate fields—behavioral ethics and behavioral economics (the latter treats deci-sions made by real, rather than ideal actors)—have concluded that the human brain has at least two modes of decision making, one of which is more appropriate for Altruistic Brain operations than the other. In *Thinking Fast and Slow*, the Nobel Prize–winning psycholo-gist Daniel Kahneman, now at Princeton, joins with the Bazerman/Tenbrunsel team's conclusion. Bazerman and Tenbrunsel want to characterize a System 1 mode of decision making as "fast, auto-matic, effortless, implicit and emotional." (Kahneman's character-ization would describe System 1 as "fast, intuitive and emotional"). In popular terms, it evokes Malcolm Gladwell's *Blink*, illustrating how intuition precipitates decision. In contrast, System 2 is "slower, conscious, effortful, explicit and more logical." (Kahneman would say: "more deliberative and more logical.") Here Bazerman and Tenbrunsel argue that if your automatic gut reaction differs from the conclusion you would reach after more deliberate System 2 cogni-tive processing, then you had better slow down and figure out exactly what that means. In particular, becoming aware of the limitations of our brain's limitations when we respond with our "wanting brains" to attractive incentives requires a degree of self-awareness essential to good, ethical decision making. The wrong circuitry produces the wrong decision.

When, because of undue speed, the wrong circuitry is used, what types of error occur? Bazerman and Tenbrunsel identify prediction errors ("what will happen if I do this...?"), and memory errors ("what have I done before, and did the results meet my standards...?"). Bernard Madoff certainly committed both types of errors. He could not have asked himself either of these questions in such a manner as to prevent his initial, thoughtless error from exploding in his face. In effect, these two experts address an error-phenomenon that implicates Step 4 of ABT, the emotionally laden neuronal switch for producing altruistic behavior. They call this phenomenon "ethical fading," such that when we make an ethical decision, details of predictions and memories of past results will fade and may already have faded, changing our motivations. This creates room for (ethical) error. As technology speeds everything up, the possibility for such errors increases accordingly.

Indeed, the first example cited by Bazerman and Tenbrunsel resonated with me because they cite the errors in manufacturing the Ford Pinto, a car that I owned. During preproduction crash tests, Ford engineers had discovered that the car's fuel tank was susceptible to rupturing, and might explode during a rear-end collision. But later, under competitive pressure from Volkswagen, Ford executives rushed toward a decision to produce the car notwithstanding the risk; perhaps they calculated that paying for the lawsuits due to passenger injury would be less expensive than a delay. In terms of ABT, the passage of time allowed for a "disconnect" between Steps 1 through 3 and Step 4. By the time they evaluated their options, the weightings had changed, especially because of Volkswagen's competitive challenge, and in Step 5 they decided to go ahead with the Pinto regardless of the possibility of fiery explosions. From a purely ethical perspective, this decision was wrong, but as Bazerman and Tenbrunsel have shown, ethics are rarely "pure."

What might a neuroscientist say to a Ford Motors executive who was standing in his study right now? First, the neuroscientist would express his humility, acknowledging a problem that is far beyond his laboratory. But then he would note that impulsive decision making interferes with Altruistic Brain mechanisms, and also that the Ford executive must think of herself as an intrinsically good person. While Altruistic Brain operations can be unconscious and fast, impulsive reflexes of the kind I am discussing preclude their proper completion. If she will simply consider the analyses of Daniel Kahneman and of our ethics experts, she will take the time to allow the "slow systems" of her brain, the so-called System 2, to operate. Memories of problems will not be lost. Prediction errors will not occur. Subsequent business decisions will be much more likely to be ethical.

In Kahneman's terms, acculturation according to "slow" as compared to "fast" modes of thinking will certainly differ among cultures. The cultures that we grow up in necessarily dominate the ways in which we are taught how to behave toward others. Obviously, cultures differ, but how? At the University of Maryland, Michelle Gelfand worked with a huge international team of researchers to study the regulation of social behaviors in 33 different nations. Her team came up with an important dichotomy: "tight" cultures, with strong norms for the regulation of social behaviors and strong sanctions against deviant behaviors, and "loose" cultures with weak norms and fewer sanctions. Two of their findings are of immediate importance. First, strict regulation of social behavior is more likely to be found in societies that are or have been exposed to major threats such as natural disasters, resource scarcity, or territorial conflict. Second, if strict adherence to religious principles bears on people's behaving well toward each other, it is good to know that "religion thrives when existential threats to human security, such as war or natural disaster, are rampant, and declines considerably in societies with high levels of economic development, low income inequality and infant mortality, and greater access to social safety nets." This kind of systematic study may help societies determine the best cultural strategies that support Altruistic Brain operations as they produce civilized behavior.

In conclusion, it seems clear that adopting Daniel Kahneman's "slow mode" of thinking and Bazerman and Tenbrunsel's "System 2" will allow the Altruistic Brain mechanism a much better chance to work. In fact, let's do a thought experiment, using a recent report on kidney donation chains in the *New York Times*. One woman in the donor chain reported that she had fleetingly considered reneging on a donation after her husband had received a donation, but that she swatted away the temptation moments later. "I believe in karma," she said, "and that would have been some really bad karma. There was somebody out there who needed my kidney." So what happened? The woman allowed her System 2 thought process to prevail, and hence she avoided a "prediction error." That is, she took time to imagine what could have happened had she failed to fulfill her commitment (some needy person would go without a kidney), and she decided against allowing that to occur. She prevented her "want brain" from overtaking her "should brain," slowing down her response to self-centered desire just enough to allow her Altruistic Brain mechanism to prevail. Unquestionably, we've all got stories like this somewhere in our memories, precisely because the potential for altruism is so strong. We just need to give it a chance, and clear away impulses that might be holding it back.

PERSPECTIVE

Understanding the neuroscience of antisocial behavior can lead to ways of avoiding such behavior and, consequently, of reinforcing our better instincts, that is, allowing our Altruistic Brain mechanisms to operate properly. Of course, though we all have the potential to act with decency, most of the problems illustrated in this chapter derive from bad individual behavior. But such bad behavior can be exacerbated, and things can get a lot worse when unfortunate individual tendencies are multiplied by individuals' participation in antisocial groups. Peer pressure can be irresistible. At-risk youngsters will tip over into gang wars. On the same trajectory, if one Nazi makes trouble, a bunch of them can make World War II. The next chapter will discuss the effect of scale—that is, of human interaction—on how bad tendencies can become really bad, large-scale actions. It will also propose approaches to how we can address this effect.

FURTHER READING

H. Anckarsater. 2006. "Central Nervous Changes in Social Dysfunction: Autism, Aggression and Psychopathy." *Brain Research Bulletin* 69, 259–265.

S. Baron-Cohen. 2011. *The Science of Evil*. New York: Basic Books.

M. Bazerman and A. Tenbrunsel. 2012. *Blind Spots*. Princeton, NJ: Princeton University Press.

Peter A. Bos, David Terburg, and Jack van Honk. 2010. "Testosterone Decreases Trust in Socially Naïve Humans." PNAS 107, 1991–1995.

W. T. Boyce. "Social Stratification, Health and Violence in the Very Young." *Annals of the New York Academy of Sciences* 1036, 47–68.

H. A. Chapman, D. A. Kim, J. M. Susskind, and A. K. Anderson, 2009. "In Bad Taste: Evidence for the Oral Origins of Moral Disgust." *Science* 323, 1222–1226.

A. D. Craig. 2009. "How Do You Feel, Now? The Anterior Insula and Human Awareness." *Nature Reviews Neuroscience* 10, 59–70.

Richard Davidson. 2012. *The Emotional Life of Your Brain*. New York: Penguin Group.

K. Dutton 2012. "The Wisdom of Psychopaths." *Scientific American* 103, 76–79.

C. Eisenegger, J. Haushofer, and E. Fehr. 2011. "The Role of Testosterone in Social Interaction." *Trends in Cognitive Science* 15, 263–270.

D. Fry. 2007. *Beyond War*. Oxford: Oxford University Press.

D. Kahneman. 2011. *Thinking Fast and Slow*. New York: Farrar, Straus and Giroux.

D. Kahneman and A. Tversky. 2000. *Choices, Values and Frames*. Cambridge, UK: Cambridge University Press.

Raymond Kelly. 2000. *Warless Societies and the Origin of War*. Ann Arbor: University of Michigan Press.

Kent A. Kiehl, Andra M. Smith, Robert D. Hare, Adrianna Mendrek, Bruce B. Forster, Johann Brink, and Peter F. Liddle. 2001. "Limbic Abnormalities in Affective Processing by Criminal Psychopaths as Revealed by Functional Magnetic Resonance Imaging." *Biological Psychiatry* 50, 677–684.

V. Menon. 2011. "Large Scale Brain Networks and Psychopathology." *Trends in Cognitive Science* 15, 483–506.

Donald Pfaff. 2011. *Man and Woman: An Inside Story*. Oxford: Oxford University Press.

Paul Rozin, J. Haidt, and C. R. McCauley. 1993. "Disgust." In M. Lewis and J. Haviland, eds., *Handbook of Emotions*, pp. 575–594. New York: Guilford.

Paul Rozin, J. Haidt, and K. Fincher. 2009. "From Oral to Moral." *Science* 323, 1179–1180.

Paul Rozin, L. Lowery, S. Imada, and J. Haidt. 1999. "The CAD Triad Hypothesis." *Journal of Personality and Social Psychology* 76, 574–589.

K. Schenck-Guftasson, P. R. DeCola, D. W. Pfaff, D. S. Pisetsky. 2012. *Handbook of Clinical Gender Medicine*. Basel: Karger.

B. Smuts. 1987. "Gender, Aggression and Influence." In B. Smut, Dorothy L. Cheney Robert M. Seyfarth, Richard W. Wrangham, and Thomas T. Struhsaker, eds., *Primate Societies*, pp. 400–412. Chicago: University of Chicago Press.

[8]

MULTIPLIER EFFECT

From Bad to Worse in a Social Setting

It must be admitted that however powerful Altruistic Brain mechanisms may be, they can be overwhelmed in some circumstances. In the previous chapter I dealt with some examples of bad behavior, but I must say that pernicious influences of groups can make it even harder to behave well. That is, Altruistic Brain mechanisms do not operate in isolation. They are beset by and must resist tendencies toward antisocial behaviors. This resistance becomes more difficult if environmental influences strengthen a person's antisocial impulses. Because "it's a tough world out there," it is important to consider some of the large-scale influences that interfere with the Altruistic Brain. That is, if it is difficult to overcome temptations presented to an individual operating *as* an individual—without any reinforcement or peer pressure—how much harder is this when bad influences are presented by powerful groups? Three types of harmful group activities have consistently engaged social scientists: gangs, war, and genocide. In this chapter, I examine how we can use Altruistic Brain Theory (ABT) to understand some of the negative group dynamics responsible for these phenomena.

GANGS

One powerful social force inhibiting the Altruistic Brain is the youth gang phenomenon. Gangs exacerbate behavioral problems in young men by permitting their peers to provide affirmation for their most aggressive tendencies. Predictably, young men join gangs in their adolescence as their testosterone begins to kick in. Once they have established themselves in a gang, members are reciprocally altruistic, perversely applying Altruistic Brain principles to cover for each other: "You take care of me. I'll watch your back." Though society cringes at the result, such baleful reciprocity makes sense from the perspective of hyped teenagers looking for support. On a much smaller scale, but increasingly, young women are also forming gangs—not in response to testosterone, of course, but to find their own communities and because young men set the example. Even more commonly, girls will form cliques, but neurobiologists have a longer history of studying instincts that lead to gang formation and gang behaviors in boys.

The data supporting my argument in this chapter have been reviewed by a social worker recommended by the New York Police Department (NYPD) anti-gang unit, and by a young man who had formerly been a gang leader but who turned his life around. These people have on-the-ground experience with the phenomena that I discuss. My point is to show that technical neuroscience can be applied to actual social problems that, until now, may have seemed intractable.

Young men join gangs in part because gangs often reproduce the members' national backgrounds; immigrants, for example, find in gangs safe havens that acknowledge their own language and culture. In *West Side Story*, Leonard Bernstein's classic musical, a Puerto Rican gang challenges a gang of English speakers, perhaps from an Irish background. (A recent Broadway revival put some dialogue into Spanish to accentuate the cultural divide.) A similar pattern prevails in gangs organized around minority ethnicities (though often ethnicity and national background converge). In different urban areas, gangs comprise diverse immigrant groups: Russians in New York, Italians in Philadelphia, Cambodians and Vietnamese in Los Angeles, and Chinese in Chinatowns around the United States. In all these cases, young men from newly arrived minority groups, isolated by language and customs from the larger society, band together for understanding, "protection," and what they perceive as a fast track to opportunity. Through their gangs, members gain access to drugs, alcohol, guns, and money. Where there is a large number of school dropouts and high unemployment, gang numbers swell. In a vicious circle, gangs encourage school drop-outs, and school drop-outs lead to gang membership. For these young people, idleness leads to crime.

Gang operations have major impacts on life in large cities because of their criminal activities. Gangs fight over territory, money, women, drugs, and just to settle old scores. And the higher street-gang density in large American cities leads to more homicides. A recent Chicago tally found 66 gangs in the city itself. The *New York Times* reported that according to Chicago police, "500 monitored gang factions have fractured into more than 600, many of them with stunningly ready access to guns." Gang members almost never come from rich families, so young boys, taught by their more experienced elders in the gangs, share in the spoils of whatever criminal activities the gang does, from simple burglaries to drug dealing. Besides gaining access to money, gang members can get guns, drugs, and alcohol. For example, among boys in Atlanta who began alcohol use before the age of 13, significantly more were gang members than non-members.

Boys who showed problematic behavior early in life, who were marginalized at school and showed low academic performance, were much more likely to join gangs around the ages of 11 or 12, according to a NYPD anti-gang unit. In turn, gang membership predicted violent behaviors by ages 18 or19. Violence spreads through every aspect of a young man's life. Once a boy joins a gang and engages in violent behavior, he is more likely to be violent, sooner or later, to his intimate partner. In well-organized studies, psychiatrists and psychologists have documented that gang membership facilitates many kinds of deviant behaviors. Boys witness violence and then participate in violence; especially vulnerable are boys with an impulsive streak and low intelligence. Indeed, scholars around the world have pointed out similarities in gang formation, always emphasizing poor neighborhoods.

So how do we reinforce Altruistic Brain operations in a manner that interferes with the effect of gangs on at-risk boys' behavior? Clearly, civic institutions must offer boys an array of outlets that substitute for potential gang membership before too much testosterone powers up a boy's brain. What about after-school games or clubs; job training; or even the opportunity to feel pride in planting trees, raising bees, or helping the homeless? What about giving kids a sense of belonging—a sense of identity—in which the group offers a safe haven, complete with familiar customs and even initiations that impart a sense of specialness? What about something as simple as curfews, which give kids a sense of limits? Any such efforts present a challenge, given the current state of austerity and the ever-available option to send youngsters away for "reform." There is a conviction among skeptics that we have tried so much, with only minimal success. But often we fail because we wait too long. If we intervene before boys' sexual and aggressive tendencies reach their full maturity—and interpose a much higher barrier to any of society's attempts at rescue—we could still have a chance.

The NYPD has a Gang Intelligence Unit that seeks to prevent gang activities that lead to major crimes. Though there is no substitute for police on the beat being familiar with the action in their assigned neighborhoods, the NYPD goes much further. It conducts surveillance on gangs by every means possible. For example, the *New York Daily News* reported that when the Unit learned that the Crips gang was using Twitter to meet up in a Brooklyn park, the police broke up the event before any violence occurred. Police monitor gangs' Facebook sites, so when gang members post reports of their criminal activities, the gang members get arrested.

Well beyond the tactics of the NYPD, I think that the problem of urban gangs is not insoluble. Some argue that gang-identified youth can be approached, for example, with respect to their health care needs. Others talk about "building relationships and resilience for the prevention of youth violence." Proactive education, with anti-gang and substitute social groups using all means of communication— assemblies, newsletters, radio, and television can, in the *ensemble*— will communicate anti-violence messages. Gang entry represents a further development on the trajectory of conduct disorders among boys who have displayed conduct disorders already. Cutting off the descent into criminality at an early stage should, correspondingly, reduce gang membership and thus gang violence.

All the means of reinforcing Altruistic Brain responses discussed in the preceding chapters could apply here because gang violence rapidly escalates, ensnaring individuals as part of a group and as part of group-on-group violence. One violent act precipitates the next, in a cycle of retaliation and counter-retaliation. Individual violent acts are not confined to the immediate victims, but ramify outwards, implicating allies of both perpetrator and victim. According to Andrew Papachristos, "individual murders between gangs create an institutionalized network of group conflict.... Murders spread through an epidemic-like process of social contagion...." That is, when a member of Gang A murders a member of Gang B, revenge by Gang B becomes obligatory, leading to a back-and-forth that has no theoretical terminus until everybody is dead. The effect is to institutionalize violence.

The fact that types of gang warfare can persist for centuries, and that as a phenomenon such hostility reveals an ancient lineage, demonstrates the perverse internal dynamics of gangs, where each member "sticks up" for the other on account of Altruistic Brain imperatives. Think, for example, of the thuggish retaliation among Shiite and Sunni gangs, which has lasted for centuries since each sect split off from the other. Or how about the Montagues and the Capulets in Shakespeare's *Romeo and Juliet*? The families were already sworn enemies as the play opens with a street brawl between them; they do not reconcile until the tragic suicides of the young lovers. Closer to home, there are the Hatfields and McCoys, whose famous feud (1863–1891) has entered the lexicon as a symbol for endless bitter rivalry sparked by honor, justice, and revenge. The recent *New York Times* article on Chicago gangs cited fights over "old grudges."

Like the example of corruption that I discussed in Chapter 6, gangs allow us to recognize that ABT can swing either way—for good or for ill—and that we can sometimes find ourselves fighting one manifestation of ABT (corruption or gangs) with another (the desire to shape up and do the socially "right" thing). This is why social action against bad outcrops such as corruption and gangs is so hard: the brain is already in a mode that seems right, and must somehow be pulled to utilize the same mechanisms to recognize a different set of right principles. No one ever said this would be easy, as the persistence of gang warfare makes clear. In many cases, gang members never leave the *culture* of gangs, but in effect "graduate" from street gangs to groups such as drug cartels, which viciously guard their territories from outsiders.

Another example of organized antisocial behavior—on a larger, even more violent scale—is war.

WAR

Theories of how war comes about have varied from discussion of tribal instincts, some inherited from nonhuman primates, to blood lust, to socioeconomic calculations. In *The Righteous Mind*, John Haidt argues that "we evolved to be tribal," and that tribes are not so much defined by the economic benefits of belonging as they are by myths and stories, narratives that Haidt calls "sacred." Requirements of how we should behave as members of a close-knit group predominate over non-group–related considerations. This is why nations "rally 'round the flag" almost reflexively. It is why the symbols and music in Leni Riefenstahl's films had such an impact, appealing to Germans' primitive love of the Fatherland, notwithstanding Hitler's atrocities. It is why Riefenstahl was Hitler's favorite filmmaker. In Haidt's words, with reference to these most primitive responses, the group's "morality blinds and binds." It is why against all the evidence to the contrary, Japan had the will to wage war in the Pacific against the United States.

Harvard biologist Richard Wrangham argues that warfare is not a unique human activity. Chimpanzees are well known to kill chimpanzees from neighboring groups. For example, near the borderline between two groups' territories, if a group of three chimps from one group sights a lone chimp on the other side, then attack, murder, and the consequent reaping of spoils and enlargement of territory may follow. The implication is that humans have "inherited" some of our warlike tendencies from chimps, such that for Wrangham, chimpanzees provide "surprisingly excellent models of our direct ancestors." Accordingly, it is possible that forms of violence exhibited by other nonhuman primates continued through the evolution of our species.

Indeed, scholars who want to argue that certain human behavioral traits find precedents in chimpanzees look for isolated early human groups that have not been touched by current social practices. Wrangham highlights a tribe called the Yanomamo as an example of a transitional group that he thinks have been "remarkably protected from modern political influences." For them, "primitive war can be deadly." Living in southern Venezuela and northern Brazil, Yanomamo people are "famous for their intense warfare." "Perpetual intervillage warfare" has been documented. Men who duck out of a war party "risk becoming known as cowards, and having their wives considered fair game for seduction." Among several other tribes cited by Wrangham, deaths due to violence ranged in his estimate from about 19 to 28%. These are the kinds of early human wars that Wrangham and other anthropologists would like to link back to chimpanzee violence. Thus, Altruistic Brain mechanisms may have a lot of inherited tendencies to overcome.

Indeed, in *Demonic Males*, Wrangham states that "chimpanzees and humans have similar patterns of violence." His argument rests, in part, on the idea that men can be violent "by temperament," that is, naturally violent. Of course, the effect of testosterone on neurons in the forebrain that are related to aggression explains some of this male aggression. In war, two features of modern military operations make it even easier to kill, whether we are talking about male or female soldiers. First, as the Nobel Prize–winning biologist Konrad Lorenz observed, long-distance weapons can make it impossible for the soldier to see his or her human target, thus removing a disincentive to killing. Second, powerful weapons that are triggered simply by a soldier's fingers do not depend on massive upper body strength. Women and small men can operate them as easily as larger, muscular soldiers. Thus, from the point of view of physical possibility, antiwar measures have more opposition than ever. The possibility of destruction by war goes beyond what Richard Wrangham even imagined.

Other thinkers also emphasize the lower, instinctual bases of war. Archeological finds of ancient massacres suggest flares of violence as soon as cities were formed. Barbara Ehrenreich has written for decades about the effect of biology on social activity. In *Blood Rites*, she argues that humans' predilection for war derives in part from their having been a small, slow, and weak species on a planet filled with large, fast, and strong predators. Not only did humans have to band together to defend themselves, she says, but as a form of social communication and bonding they celebrated "blood rites," whose ceremonies reenacted the terrifying experiences of dealing with such predators.

But how does Ehrenreich get from early human ceremonies around the communal fire to modern war and genocide? First, she reminds us that predation by large carnivores persisted until not so long ago. Tigers terrorized Indian villages into the 20th century. In more general terms, Ehrenreich bridges the gap from ancient blood rites to recent wars by deriving from such rites the basis of modern, communally sanctioned, socially organized violence.

Ehrenreich's reasoning for how we got to modern genocide begins with the recognition that in the history of humankind, some individuals were and are much more capable of carrying out violent acts than others. Large, strong males obviously were the best candidate, and from their choice there evolved "warrior elites." Out of "work" much of the time, they tried to ensure their own survival within society by attempting to invest their roles as "sacred and worthy of general respect." Ehrenreich posits that in some cases these groups of male warriors further "gained religious legitimacy" by arranging for tribute from their vanquished foes, not just in the form of looted goods but also "in the form of human sacrificial material."

Ehrenreich brings examples from all around the world, but focuses on three cases of "war worship": Nazism, as manifest in Germany during the 1930s and 1940s; Japanese Shintoism, during the early part of the 20th century; and extreme forms of American patriotism right now, which under circumstances of war can "evoke bursts of nationalist religiosity." In these and other cases, threats from outsiders to the nations in question stimulate defensive reactions that have a religious character such that warrior leaders might actually be worshiped.

In such examples, manifest across our planet, people behave exactly as predicted by ABT: they bond with and protect each other, even if in doing so they produce mayhem. In Ehrenreich's words "they enjoy the company of their fellows and thrill to the prospect of joining them in collective defense against the common enemy." That is, people are willing to put out extreme effort and to suffer the risk of injury and death, in order to protect the interests of others who belong to the same collective as they do.

War would seem easier than ever now, for two reasons. First, consider the point made by Konrad Lorenz. In dramatic contrast with medieval hand-to-hand fighting, today's soldiers usually can see, up close and personal, the people whom they are about to kill. What does that do to the attitudes and emotions of the aggressor? Second, though in human history, virtually all of the combatants have been male, now female soldiers can operate complicated military equipment quite as well as men. As more and more commanders and other influential leaders are female, strategic choices—especially those centering on whether to initiate aggressive acts or not—could change.

Thus when Altruistic Brain processes are activated, and people are in an environment that fosters the formation of gangs or wars, social forces within their social units make it especially easy for violent behavior to occur. From the moment that a soldier enters boot camp, he is trained to depersonalize, indeed dehumanize other men—men who are collectively labeled The Enemy. Such training suppresses Altruistic Brain processes and allows men's most aggressive tendencies to become their default drive. Of course, within gangs or a group of soldiers in a foxhole, the camaraderie encourages altruistic behavior. Think of *Saving Private Ryan*. In a foxhole you are fiercely dedicated to protecting your buddy, and you know that he will do the same for you. Altruistic Brain processes work within the context of a fighting unit—they make the "unit" possible—even though we recognize that the formation of gangs and prosecution of wars issues in undesirable mass violence.

None of these anthropological and biological theories of war are mutually exclusive. They could all have been operating in human history and all could be operating today. Nor do such biological approaches deny the cogency of cool, calculated economic and historical thinking. The Prussian officer Carl von Clausewitz, a widely recognized theorist of war, observed that war is "a continuation of policy by other means." In other words, war can be a rational undertaking. Even as the historian Barbara Tuchman emphasized "the loss of rational thought in the service of political folly," other historians, notably Yale's Donald Kagan, look at political factors that vary according to the period, the country, and the war.

Kagan and other historians know that well beyond "biological" theories of war, groups of humans operating at high levels of organization and cognition make strategic calculations and mistakes that can lead to war. In *Origins of War*, Kagan explores this phenomenon in four wars, two ancient and two modern. For example, with respect to the Peloponnesian War between Athens and Sparta, Kagan denied the claim by the ancient Greek historian Thucydides that war was an inevitable result of the growth of the Athenian empire. Instead, Kagan described a reasoned calculation by the Athenians concerning the predicted behavior of their allies, the Corinthians. Their calculations were wrong, and by accident the Corinthians provoked the Spartans, who therefore launched an attack on the Corinthians and the Athenians. Kagan concludes that a miscalculation led the Athenians into a war that they had been trying to avoid. Kagan makes an analogy to the run-up to World War I. At that time, Germany was a strong military power, dissatisfied with its status in Europe. The British could have avoided the horrendous bloodbath of World War I if they had had the foresight to establish strong, well-publicized military alliances with France and Russia. By miscalculating, they failed to do so and, in turn, failed to achieve deterrence of Germany and were sunk into World War I. Those two cases, one ancient and one modern, are examples of miscalculations.

Other examples, both ancient and modern, show war due to simple inaction. To quote Kagan, "No peace keeps itself." The Second Punic War was set up by Roman inaction. Rome, having won the

First Punic War, failed to ratify a reasonable treaty with Hannibal and Carthage. Hannibal attacked an important Roman base in Spain, and it took Rome more than a year to respond, thus giving Hannibal time to invade Italy. Kagan says that Rome was then forced "to pay the price of a long, blood, costly, devastating and almost fatal war." A parallel can be found in World War II. European democracies, so affected by the horrors of World War I, held "blind hope that a refusal to contemplate war... would somehow keep the peace." Had these democracies taken action to effectively and visibly prepare for war, German generals might not have followed Hitler's overly ambitious plans for conquest.

Many historical thinkers would claim that wars and even attempts at genocide do not simply "break out," but are instead planned, that they are based on longstanding social fears, and are timed rationally for maximum political gain and minimum negative consequences. Moreover, it is disputed whether ancestral human societies were primarily peaceful or primarily warlike. But computer modeling based on estimates of the levels of mortality consequent to intergroup violence suggests that extensive lethal conflicts would have killed off enough warlike participants as to "affect the evolution of human social behaviors," thus promoting prosocial behaviors beneficial to early human groups.

Indeed, as University of Washington psychology professor David Barash argues, war is a recent phenomenon in the life of the human species. That is, it is not part of our evolutionary inheritance. In a recent article, "Is There a War Instinct?," Barash takes issue with scholars who generalize from a few warlike tribes (notably the Yanomami) to all of humanity, and states that war is historically contingent, not biologically compelled:

> A useful distinction in this regard is between evolved *adaptations* and *capacities*. Language is almost certainly an *adaptation*, something that all normal human beings can do, although the details vary

with circumstance. By contrast, reading and writing are *capacities*, derivative traits that are unlikely to have been directly selected for, but have developed through cultural processes. Similarly, walking and probably running are adaptations; doing cartwheels or handstands are capacities. In my view, interpersonal violence is a human adaptation, not unlike sexual activity, parental care, communication and so forth. It is something we see in every human society. Meanwhile, war—being historically recent, as well as erratic in worldwide distribution and variation in detail—is almost certainly a capacity. And capacities are neither universal or mandatory.

Barash's argument fits with my own in that he situates war as a response to factors outside and subsequent to the species' evolutionary development. He even takes Steven Pinker to task for citing the decline of war while assuming that it "'characterized life in a state of nature.'" Barash presses his argument—as do I—out of a conviction that how we think about war, that is, how we think about human nature, influences how we determine our political and cultural priorities. He asks: "How many arms races and cycles of international distrust have been fed by a pre-existing view that the other side is aggressive, potentially violent and irremediably warlike, which in turn leads to policies and actions that further confirm such assumptions?" By dispelling an unfortunate misapprehension about the human species, premised on insufficient empirical research, Barash clears a space in the discourse for a science-based discussion of the psychology of war.

To develop such a discourse, this book makes an initial effort to suggest how Altruistic Brain operations could be strengthened and, hopefully, how one's knowledge of one's own moral circuitry can help in that regard. Academic efforts of this sort might help to dispel violence. But specifically with regard to war, how could society organize to discourage it? Many thinkers have stated that by educating women more extensively and providing career paths to power, we could go a long way toward reducing the incidence of war. This is because women—unlike men—are not governed by testosterone.

To quote the American psychiatrist David Hamburg, "Our species has a long history of distrusting strangers, despising outgroups and fighting each other in many ways and many places, using the most damaging technology available at the time." But human beings can proceed without war. If war is not inevitable, then social scientists must do a better job of describing the social and economic factors that discourage warfare. In ancient times, tribal aggressiveness was fierce, as shown by archeological evidence of mass slaughters, but some ancient tribes have carried on without war. The anthropologist Douglas Fry cites a considerable number of examples of warless societies that have persisted, from aboriginal Australians to the tribes of India's Nilgiri and Wynaad plateaus, to the semi-nomadic hunter-gatherer peoples of the Labrador Peninsula in Canada. Modern Switzerland and Costa Rica provide current examples of nations that have stayed out of wars. Hopefully, these small countries will provide examples for their larger counterparts.

Believing in the biological determinism of war—that humans' natural aggression leads, naturally and inevitably to war—is itself harmful. While sociologists and anthropologists have concentrated on social structures in society that they hypothesize will militate against war, every society is composed of individuals who make decisions, and those decisions do not necessarily conform to the demands of (militaristic) groups. Individual knowledge of Altruistic Brain circuitry should help individuals to make decisions that contribute to the modern decline in organized violence. That is, people who accept the fact that their brains are wired with Altruistic Brain circuitry, and that the presumed targets of their potentially violent behavior are comparably wired, will be less likely to contemplate violence. In fact, the decline was recently documented by Steven Pinker (albeit he assumed that warlike behavior was part of human nature). Altruistic instincts, prominent in our primate relatives like bonobos, have persisted in humans' history, can easily work according to brain mechanisms described in Chapter 4, and should be encouraged. How we can use social tools to strengthen the altruistic tendency is discussed in the last chapter.

GENOCIDE

Throughout human history, large groups of people have committed genocide—mass atrocities, including attempts to exterminate entire races or nations. While sheer hatred and long-simmering religious or tribal animosity is often the proximate motivation for such acts, many experts believe that the perpetrators also have unstated political or economic goals, including a lust for additional land and resources. For example, Alex De Waal of Tufts University argues that efforts to deter genocide "tend to misconstrue or overlook the fundamental motivations of the perpetrators," and that while racial causes may provide a justification, "most mass killers have other goals." De Waal observes that during the Nigerian civil war of the 1960s, military leaders, having achieved a necessary but limited victory, "began a process of reconciliation and reconstruction under the banner 'no victor, no vanquished.'" They did not *want* to continue the killing, even though they could have. Their main goal was to gain and hold power, not just to wipe out potential rivals; when that goal was reached there was no further reason for more slaughter. Speaking to this type of situation, in which there are apparently ulterior motives, De Waal notes that "The killers usually have political goals: They are determined to kill until they achieve their objectives." Note the word "until:" if the main purpose is not simply killing for its own sake— that is, not simply killing to wipe out every so-called enemy—then the killing no longer serves any purpose and will just stop.

So here is the key point. Recognizing the political/economic goals of would-be mass murderers creates a natural opening for negotiation. As Daniel Kahneman would say, "slow down, let's think about this." Negotiations that halt the rush to war permit the parties to pursue nondestructive social processes. As Winston Churchill is reported to have told a White House meeting in 1954, "It is better to jaw-jaw than to war-war." Of course, even if people do agree to slow down and talk, they still need some reason to keep talking, and not to walk away because they would *rather* fight than risk losing what they think they can ultimately obtain (albeit at some cost to themselves). This is where ABT comes in. Recognition of everyone's Altruistic Brain capacities could encourage the perpetrators to appreciate that their intended victims are not just means to an end, but rather people with comparable needs and desires. *They are people with whom one may be able to develop trust.* At this point, the talking could begin—or at least what diplomats call "talks about talks," those preliminary negotiations about procedures and protocols. Behind these "talks" there should come frank discussions based on developing a workable, hopefully durable trust. Once it seems to be established, then if the real reasons for hostilities are to acquire land and resources, economists and agronomists from both sides could initiate practical talks, perhaps long-term agreements that open up lands to leasing and make resources available at fair, even mutually beneficial long-term prices. Partnership is often cheaper in the long run than war, and it will be up to the parties to ensure that in their case this is so. For each conflict, each conversation will be different. But there will also be a common substrate: ABT can, and ideally should give the parties assurance that if they sit down with potential opponents they will be able to talk long enough to reach some *modus vivendi*.

Of course, the challenges will be immense. At a July, 2012 symposium on how to avert future genocide, Yale professor Timothy Snyder argued that climate change will act as a "multiplier of other resource crises," causing uncertainty about resources and an "ecological panic that I'm afraid will lead to mass killings in the decades to come." This panic, he said, has in fact already started, as the United States and China scramble for resources (including such basics as food) and thereby destabilize the resource bases of other countries. Though then Secretary of State Hillary Clinton said that governments must galvanize their efforts to prevent genocide, how can such "efforts" coexist with efforts by these same governments to feed their people, find water, and maintain access to supplies of energy? And what happens when climate change exacerbates the effect of population increases in countries already under stress? Will they be pushed over the edge toward even sooner than they might otherwise be from outside pressure? It may be that we cannot wait for the next crisis to develop, and that useful talks might begin now to integrate Altruistic Brain assumptions into long-term, equitable planning.

LESSONS LEARNED

In several types of social organizations, Altruistic Brain mechanisms face massive opposition from the desire to join gangs, make war, or even to commit genocide. Opportunities to overcome the motives for such action arise when we recognize that individuals joining gangs or planning wars usually have identifiable rationales that, on reflection, might be peacefully addressed. That is, switching from fast, impulsive thinking to Kahneman's more considered "thinking slow" may give Benevolent Brain mechanisms a chance to work. Further encouragement in the belief that we can bolster the Benevolent Brain comes in the next chapter.

I appreciate that there are skeptics, indeed very fine academics, who dismiss the idea that hard-core neurobiology can point the way toward so complex a concept as moral behavior. But the ideas that I have discussed in this chapter are modest, and, of course, I am not trying to speak as a social scientist. Instead, as a neuroscientist I am trying to offer a new way of understanding how individuals engage with each other. This understanding must, of course, be refracted through all of the circumstances to which individuals and groups react. But it can nonetheless encourage us to think that we can mitigate the effects of some of the toughest circumstances. If we think that there are demonstrable bases to act positively in groups, then perhaps there is a greater chance that we will.

FURTHER READING

David Barash. 2013, September 19. "Is There a War Instinct?" *Aeon* http://www.aeon-magazine.com/living-together/human-beings-do-not-have-an-instinct-for-war/

S. Bowles. 2009. "Did Warfare among Ancestral Hunter-gatherers Affect the Evolution of Human Social Behaviors?" *Science* 324, 1293–1299.

Barbara Ehrenreich. 1997. *Blood Rites: Origin and History of the Passions of War.* New York: Metropolitan Books.

Douglas Fry. 2007. *Beyond War: The Human Potential for Peace.* Oxford: Oxford University Press.

Douglas Fry. 2012. "Life without War." *Science* 336, 879–884.

Jonathan Haidt. 2012. *The Righteous Mind.* New York: Pantheon.

J. Horgan. 2012. *The End of War.* San Francisco: McSweeny's Books.

Donald Kagan. 1995. *On the Origins of War and the Preservation of Peace.* New York: Doubleday.

A. Papachristos. 2009. "Murder by Structure: Dominance Relations and the Social Structure of Gang Homicide." *American Journal of Sociology* 115, 74–128.

Donald Pfaff. 2007. *Neuroscience of Fair Play.* New York: Dana Press.

D. Stapel and S. Lindenberg. 2011. "Coping with Chaos: How Disordered Contexts Promote Stereotyping and Discrimination." *Science* 332, 251–255.

Barbara Tuchman. 1985. *The March of Folly: From Troy to Vietnam.* New York: Ballantine Books.

Richard Wrangham. 1999. "Evolution of Coalitionary Killing." *Yearbook of Physical Anthropology* 42, 1–30.

Richard Wrangham and D. Peterson. 1996. *Demonic Males: Apes and the Origins of Human Violence.* Boston: Houghton-Mifflin.

[9]

NO EASY ANSWERS . . . BUT
NO PESSIMISM EITHER

If Altruistic Brain Theory (ABT) is an accurate description of how humans behave altruistically, then how can our common neural circuitry provide a means for encouraging such behavior? This chapter presents ways to approaches this question.

The Altruistic Brain offers evidence that based on our neural circuitry, we can believe in our own good nature. It argues further that such belief can have positive, even transformative effects in individual lives. But now let's take this concept to the next level: in mathematical terms, imagine the Altruistic Brain Squared. That is, what if each person's belief in himself were generalized within a social setting or particular group, such that everyone in that group believed in everyone else's good nature? This could produce an altruistic "multiplier effect," the obverse of that baleful effect discussed in Chapter 8. Thus instead of a mass of bad people, each making the other behave even worse, groups of good people would synergize each other's best inclinations. This chapter proposes some ideas for how to encourage this effect.

Specifically, it will suggest means whereby society can institutionalize individual altruistic inclinations, so that they become part of the social fabric. In a nutshell, knowing that our brains are wired for good behavior now makes it possible to chart (and promote) the consequences of such wiring for our behavior in groups. Think about it: the armed forces depend on an *esprit de corps* where the trust—even love—that troops feel toward each other help make a tough mission possible. The more that men in a unit get to know each other and appreciate each other's value, the more each is willing to share the sacrifices that combat entails. The unit begins to act *as* a unit. The same is true in business settings, where late-night "bull" sessions help to humanize co-workers, making a difficult project more of a commitment than a task (this is why companies encourage outings, picnics, volleyball teams, and even group cooking classes). Indeed, speaking of sports, we have all seen how after a winning game, the players tend to jump up and hug one another, acknowledging that the win would have been impossible without the synergy of a lot of good men (or women). In this same vein, ER doctors, nurses, and paramedics pull together, instinctively relying on each other, working as a *team* to help injured patients survive a trauma. And of course there are firemen, who beyond their training develop loyalties that allow them to provide mutual support under tremendous stress. (Just think back to our discussion of Steven Siller, in Chapters 2 and 3, who was motivated, in part, by envisioning the pain of his buddies already at the scene). Indeed, life is full of examples of positive "group-think," in which members of the group understand how their mutual high regard allowed each to cooperate with and rely on the other, producing a positive outcome.

As Stephen Post has suggested, one version of this group-think is found in organizations with a "positive hierarchy," where reciprocity is expected, exhorted, acknowledged, and rewarded. Within such organizations, an ethos of service emanates from the top down; it permeates the organization, and no one is allowed to forget that each person is responsible for the success of its efforts. Thus there are good reasons why the Army bestows Purple Hearts and Bronze Stars. Beyond their recognition of the individual recipients, such medals are powerful symbols of the organization's values, and help to reinforce them.

Of course, there are no easy answers to longstanding social problems, and I do not claim that neuroscience provides a magic bullet. We must resist reductive, one-size-fits-all solutions. However, ABT is naturally compatible with two types of social strategies that seem more workable on account of the theory, whether they are employed individually or in any combination:

- James Gilligan's idea that we treat concerns over moral behavior as we would a problem of public health
- The empowerment of women, lessening the effect of testosterone-driven behavior in society

The virtue of ABT is that it enhances other approaches, allowing us to understand why they are advantageous and how, in fact, we can make improve them. Acknowledging that people are diverse, and that we will never be able to go into communities with a predesigned "fix," we can still add the benefits of neuroscience to existing, proven methodologies so as to gain deeper insights into their operative principles and emphasize aspects of those principles that will work best in any given situation.

APPROACH PROMOTION OF ETHICAL BEHAVIORS AS A PUBLIC HEALTH ISSUE

Well-designed social initiatives can promote the operation of Altruistic Brain mechanisms even under difficult conditions—poverty, gang warfare, neighborhood decline. The most comprehensive framework for how society can reinforce our built-in ethical circuitry comes from James Gilligan, M.D., now professor of psychiatry at New York University. During his years at Harvard Medical School, he was Chief of Psychiatry for the Massachusetts prison system. He knows whereof he speaks.

Gilligan's program has three phases.

Phase One: Primary Prevention

"Primary [or first-level] prevention" includes strategies that target an entire cohort with preventative measures, without addressing particular, individual differences. At this level of approach, Gilligan states that we must prevent the humiliation of young boys in order to preserve their self-image from degradation. Building on this idea, we can deduce that boys' potential faith in own good inclinations needs to be supported.

Gilligan proposes that the first round of measures to encourage prosocial behavior should apply to an entire population. While in the past, measures supporting "public health" required clean water and an adequate sewer system, Gilligan uses "Primary Prevention" to mean the creation of circumstances to prevent development of structures in society that promote violence.

Reducing social and economic inequities, or ameliorating their effects, would top any list of Gilligan-type measures. Time and again, reducing the effects of "class" differences has proven more effective in preventing violent crime than relying on post-offense criminal punishment. Researchers in the United States have produced many studies on this point and, in the United Kingdom, Prof. Richard Wilkinson makes the same argument.

In this regard, ensuring that children do not go through elementary and middle school as anonymous little cogs—that is, ensuring that classes are small enough that they are recognized as real people—is crucial. This idea is taken for granted in well-to-do school districts, but it's a problem in their poorer counterparts. Current literature on brain structure and molecular genetics demonstrate the dire consequences of not providing adequate support for children, especially those from deprived backgrounds who are prone to humiliation.

It is particularly important to avoid humiliation of young boys, because they will remember it forever; when testosterone begins to flood their brains, those memories will be used to justify generalized acts of revenge. As Chapter 6 demonstrates, the robust apparatus by which testosterone facilitates aggressive behaviors stands ready to operate in every adolescent male.

Failure to implement Gilligan's Phase One principles risks causing boys to suffer the consequences of long-term changes in the brain. For example, let's think of the potential effects of damaging early experiences on boys' aggressive behavior, the kind of situation I highlighted in Chapter 8. When a boy is repeatedly put in stressful situations by shortages of basic necessities, social embarrassment, or especially by hostility within his family, two types of chemical changes can result in the neurons of his brain. Both can detrimentally alter gene expression in those neurons for a long time.

In one such chemical change (Figure 9.1), an excrescence composed of a carbon atom and three hydrogen atoms is added to a part of the brain's DNA. A team at McGill University showed the devastating effect of such changes occurring on account of early childhood abuse. They studied DNA obtained from the hippocampi (parts of

DNA Methylation

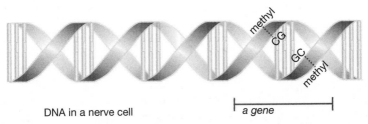

DNA in a nerve cell · a gene

Figure 9.1 An epigenetic change in the brain. Adding a chemical "decoration," a methyl group (one carbon atom, three hydrogen atoms) to a gene suppresses the expression of that gene in that nerve cell for a long time, perhaps permanently. As a result, behaviors regulated by that nerve cell can be affected permanently.

our ancient forebrain) of suicide victims with histories of such abuse. Not only was the excrescence increased, but as a result gene expression for the brain's stress hormone receptor was decreased. One could have predicted abnormal responses to stress in such individuals and, sure enough, they committed suicide.

The other chemical change occurs in histones, a part of the proteins that guard access to DNA (Figure 9.2). My Rockefeller University colleague David Allis proposes that there is a "histone code," roughly analogous to the bar code on groceries, that can be translated into a molecular formula for regulating genes. Thinking about neurons that control behavior in the brains of boys who have been damaged during development—perhaps by poverty or a violent father—it appears that permanent alterations in gene expressions have the potential to warp behavior for decades. To paraphrase another of my colleagues, Bruce McEwen, it is difficult to overestimate the power of early-life

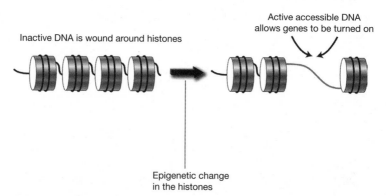

Figure 9.2 Epigenetic change: little "barrels" of histone proteins in the nerve cell nucleus keep inactive DNA wound up and inaccessible to chemicals that would turn genes on. As a result of early experience those histone proteins can be changed chemically so that the DNA gets free and the genes in the accessible DNA can be turned on. As a result, behaviors that depend on those genes can be changed permanently.

abuse and neglect to affect lifelong behavior, in that such abuse affects the health of the entire body as well as the brain.

Such molecular changes affect not only the brain's chemistry, but are likely as well to affect the structure and function of the brain. A recent study from the Washington University School of Medicine looked at the effect on the hippocampus of good maternal attention given to a group of children who suffered from depression. The hippocampus regulates much of our emotional reactions to stress, but also is essential for converting short-term memories into long-term memory. The study compared the hippocampal sizes of children four to seven years old who were given high levels of maternal support as observed under somewhat stressful hospital conditions versus children who were given low levels of maternal support. Children with high levels of maternal support had much larger hippocampal sizes. The results suggest that these children will have better functioning hippocampi during development and probably into adulthood, and most likely better memory function and reactions to stress. In effect, good treatment led to positive brain development.

Though the study focused on the positive effects of good parental care, it's important also to quote the reverse situation: that in a large number of studies with experimental animals, deficient care of the babies translated into a variety of behavioral problems, including social behavioral problems. One such study scanned the brains of participants while they participated in a computer ball-throwing game. Some participants were always included in the game, while others were excluded. The study confirmed that those latter subjects *felt* excluded. The social exclusion activated an emotionally important part of our cerebral cortex, right in the middle of our brains, that closely paralleled the activation of that cortical region by physical pain. Thus, when social conditions in a young child's life fail Gilligan's Phase One, the failing caregivers may be sentencing the child to years of cortical malfunctions that, as far as brain functions are concerned, are as severe as physical pain.

These results lead us to a substantial literature in which social realities can be found to map onto the neurological representation of physical realities, such as physical pain or reward. One such study found that even such a common, everyday experience as envy of another's success activates the same part of the cortex as physical pain does. Conversely, experiencing "illicit joy" at a competitor's misfortune activated circuitry in the forebrain associated with positive physical reward. A variety of positive social experiences map onto nerve cell activation associated with physical reward; and the reverse, ordinary social problems associated with nerve cell activation similar to pain. There is no reason to believe that success or failure, respectively, with respect to a child's experience regarding Gilligan Phase One will not be registered in this pain/pleasure circuitry for the rest of his or her life.

According to James Q. Wilson's "Broken Windows" theory of crime, once trouble begins, it spreads. Disorder and evidence of social neglect breed more of the same. In the Dutch city of Groningen, Kees Keizer set up conditions featuring graffiti, physical disorder, and inducement to stealing. Results were clear: early indications of disorder led to more disorder. Inappropriate behavior will lead to more inappropriate behavior. The success of New York City's "Quality of Life" campaign gives informal support to Keizer's results. By paying attention to things like graffiti, vandalism, and clean streets—so-called minor problems—the City actually reduced crime. More recently, the Harlem Children's Zone, founded by Geoffrey Canada, achieved notable success in literally repairing broken windows through its Community Pride program. As the Zone's website states, that program draws on the good will of community residents, who act in concert to upgrade their living conditions:

> Community Pride organizes tenant and block associations, helping many hundreds of tenants convert their city-owned buildings

into tenant-owned co-ops. The program combines social services for individuals and families with tenant organizing and community redevelopment initiatives. This comprehensive strategy allows Community Pride's staff to operate simultaneously at three levels of intervention: families, building and block. The program also works with and impacts other stakeholders such as churches and police precincts.

Community Pride's work is guided by an overall community development philosophy that is based on the participation of community residents in all planning and decision-making activities.

The value of this type of approach is that no one feels left out; concomitantly, everyone is offered the chance to shoulder responsibility, to form networks with others and to discover what they can personally contribute to the effort. The notion of "Pride," so closely linked to self-esteem, operates as a foundational principle, enabling the individual—magnified by the results achieved by the group—to feel good about his own potential. That feeling is enhanced as the "broken windows" are repaired, and the environment ceases to be an affront to any possibility of hope. Geoffrey Canada, among others, affirms that secure environments—physical and social—make it easier for prosocial, altruistic behavior to occur.

The notion that good residences make good residents is shared across the ideological spectrum. Even moderately conservative thinkers have acknowledged that that residents of tough parts of American cities have bad values. Such people "lack the social capital" to put good values into play. Social context is important. "No matter how social disorganization gets started, it takes on a momentum of its own. People who grow up in disrupted communities are more likely to lead disrupted lives as adults, magnifying disorder from one generation to the next." The point is to break the cycle.

Another way in which social programs can multiply the benefits of individual self-esteem, and hence Altruistic Brain capacity, is through what Mark Greenberg, Professor of Psychology at Penn State, calls "school-based prevention of behavioral problems and promotion of caring and competence." Interventions in schools are effective because schools play a crucial role in children's lives. One such intervention that has been highly documented is the development of curricula to "teach students new skills which build their competence to engage in positive peer and adult relations, and to develop self-control and healthy values and norms to resist engagement in deviant or dangerous behavior." These efforts, part of a multidisciplinary initiative called Social and Emotional Learning, have been reported to reduce violence and aggression, particularly in children of lower socioeconomic status; they also reduce early use of alcohol, obviously preventing a variety of behavioral problems.

In *Grand Pursuit: The Story of Economic Genius*, Sylvia Nasar argues that our social attitudes are intertwined with our economic circumstances. For the past three decades, real wages of American workers have been falling. No longer can parents feel that their children's quality of life will be better than their own. Such loss of hope threatens our society's future. It corrodes the social fabric. To restore hope and begin to build a sustainable future, we must restore the economic and social dynamic that undergirded social aspiration. While it's up to politicians, economists—and voters—with regard to how to accomplish this, it's clear that we have to.

Of course, in every developed and developing economy it is urgent to find meaningful employment for young people, especially those in large cities where crime is higher. Reinforcing what science knows about adolescents' visions of themselves, we must help them to maintain a positive vision of their roles in adult society; this will help them to maintain their positive self-image, which, in turn, will foster good behavior. In this regard, universal national service at either or both of two ages—the first pre-gang and the second post–high school—could teach vocational skills particularly important for those who don't go to college. As Harvard political scientist Robert Putnam reported, "It's perfectly understandable that kids from working-class backgrounds have become cynical and even paranoid, for virtually all our major social institutions have failed them—family, friends, church, school and community."

David Kennedy reports that he has succeeded in reducing inner-city violence in several American cities. In *Don't Shoot*, he writes that he believes in bringing together three communities: law enforcement, local family groups, and "the community of the streets (people who bond by hanging around street corners and other sleazy locales)." Young boys must be addressed personally by these communities so as to convince them to follow the law and avoid gangs. Those who engage them must have legitimacy in these boys' eyes. According to Kennedy, a simple, inexpensive, direct neighborhood commitment that says "I [the local resident] am going to STOP that [street problem] from happening" is the essence of prevention. Law enforcement, he says, must be seen as part of an overall, citizen-based effort to prevent inner-city violence.

All of these thinkers talk of broad-scale preventative measures that would, effectively, make it easier for Altruistic Brain circuitry to work effectively. But let's think outside the box for a moment. Another idea just coming to the fore is to take better control of the climate, as new research emerges on the link between extreme climate and upsurges in violence. As the journal *Science* reported in August 2013, a large meta-study tabulating results in areas as diverse as archaeology, criminology, economics, geography, history, political science, and psychology demonstrates that where temperatures increased or rainfall decreased there was a marked increase in individual and group violence. This makes sense instinctively, as we have all seen tempers flare when it's hot and we have all heard about conflicts over water in the American southwest and the Middle East. But now there is beginning to be real proof of yet another reason to conserve resources and address climate change.

Phase Two: Secondary (Targeted) Prevention

"Secondary prevention" includes preventative measures targeted at particularly high-risk individuals. Where Phase One efforts are insufficient, therefore, Gilligan states that society must marshal its resources to support young men who are behaviorally challenged, often where their environments discourage ethical behavior.

It is true that despite society's best efforts to follow Phase One recommendations, some young people will still need special attention because of their predispositions or unusual development. In these instances, the problem can be addressed using "secondary strategies" employed by public health authorities. By analogy, if we were concerned about secondary prevention of cardiovascular disease, we would pay special attention to people with a family history of this disease who are also overweight; we would seek to lower their cholesterol and blood pressure before their first heart attack or stroke. This type of intervention can be applied to behavioral problems. If parents and other authorities sense that certain children are at higher than average risk for developing antisocial behaviors, then these children should be offered programs to help head off the dangers of antisocial behaviors.

Such programs would obviously include various types of support initiatives, but they could also focus on specific problems such as the prevention of bullying. It is impossible to overstate the effects bullying with regard to humiliation and the creation of social underclasses— the bullies and the bullied. Tom Boyce, now at the University of British Columbia, shows that "social stratification" among youth contributes to violence. He suggests that under conditions conducive to bad behavior, we must pay attention to these extremes: the highest and the lowest in the dominance hierarchy. We must recognize the tendencies of the former to turn into bullies and the latter to suffer from physiological effects of prolonged stress. We must bring both extremes into a domain where Altruistic Brain mechanisms can work effectively.

The effect of sex differences on the rate of bullying is clear: boys will be more aggressive. Even though I have argued previously that many aspects of social life used to be seen as (but really aren't) exclusively men's domains, it remains true that testosterone fuels the adolescent boy's capacity for aggressive or even violent behavior. Chapter 7 spelled out molecular mechanisms and neural circuitry for these primitive behavioral effects. As a result of these effects, caregivers must remain particularly alert to identify young boys for whom acting out is going to become a major problem, and help them put their physical and mental energies to better uses. In the *New York Times*, David Brooks pointedly argued that redirecting boys' unruly energies is not the same thing as simply calming them down. Rather, he stated, we have to figure out what positive values may lurk behind all that energy, and then try to make the most of those values through a multipronged approach that recognizes individual differences:

Schools have to engage people as they are. That requires leaders who insist on more cultural diversity in school; not just teachers who celebrate cooperation, but other teachers who celebrate competition; not just teachers who honor environmental virtues, but teachers who honor military virtues; not just curriculums that teach how to share, but curriculums that teach how to win and how to lose; not just programs that work like friendship circles, but programs that work like boot camp.

The basic problem is that schools praise diversity but have become culturally homogenous. The education world has become a distinct subculture, with a distinct ethos and attracting a distinct sort of employee. Students who don't fit the ethos get left out.

Applying the logic of Brooks' argument, we can seek to create an environment for testosterone-driven boys that will provide individualized *outlets* for their own best tendencies, allowing them to conform to general notions of social usefulness even as they express their particular identities. If Altruistic Brain mechanisms push us toward the "good," it is still possible that goodness can be broadly defined, allowing for some play in the joints of social engineering. I don't even like that term, "engineering," as it tends to place the emphasis on how one group controls another. The idea is to offer multiple attractive options to children, and then let their own best impulses lead them in directions that work best for them.

But we still have to prevent raw violence, and give these optimizing measures a chance to work. Some well-organized interventions are addressing young boys whose Altruistic Brain processes are challenged by crime-ridden environments. The Interruptors, operating in the roughest neighborhoods of Chicago, "interrupt" the development of seriously aggressive, hostile encounters. The group is composed of smart young men and women who themselves grew up in similar neighborhoods, and who convince young men that they are and can be "better than that." In such an endeavor, no record could be perfect, but the group claims many successes. The Interruptors are breaking up environmental conditions that war against altruistic brain mechanisms and giving the neuronal wiring posed by ABT a greater chance to work.

Phase Three: Amelioration

"Tertiary" measures address individuals who already exhibit various forms of antisocial behavior. In such instances, Gilligan recommends that society seek to ameliorate these individuals' conditions, and if possible return them to a more hopeful state. Transposing Gilligan's schema into a neuroscience context, we must use every means possible to allow Altruistic Brain mechanisms to operate in the brains of young men who have violated the law or social norms.

It is obvious that regardless of our best efforts in Phase One and Phase Two, some children are going to get in trouble. So what do we do? Gilligan's approach would say that we are entering the domain of clinical, rather than preventive, medicine: taking care of a patient already ill to prevent the illness from becoming chronic or contagious.

Clearly, the first step will involve psychotherapy and will emphasize that this is a good person who has gone (redeemably) wrong. The patient's acceptance of his or her naturally altruistic brain mechanisms would certainly help.

Second, there should be attempts at behavioral modification, and the consequent choice between rewards offered by the therapist ("positive reinforcement") for compliant behaviors and punishments ("negative reinforcement") for continued noncompliant behavior. For many therapists, staying with positive reinforcement is the way to go. In fact, the "father" of behaviorism, B. F. Skinner, frowned on the use of negative reinforcement because of the harmful responses to punishment that impede the patient's learning process.

In *SuperCooperators*, Harvard's Martin Nowak supports Gilligan's (and Skinner's) opposition to "negative reinforcement." Nowak and his students used computers to stage competitions among programs that deployed what they called "evolutionary game theory." Ethical standards were built into the games, which included more than 1000 interactions among pairs of players. The main goal was to evaluate the role of punishment following unethical behavior in the game. Strikingly, none of the six best-performing players ever used punishment to correct unethical behavior. The worst-performing players, however, used punishment most often. Punishment evidently interferes with the smooth operation of Altruistic Brain processes, but the exact mechanisms by which this interference occurs are still to be discovered.

Therapies that utilize psychotropic drugs may at some point be integrated with policies and programs for helping patients avoid anti-social behavior. The combined efforts of government-funded research in the United States and abroad has produced large numbers of drugs for a wide range of behavioral disorders. The object, ideally, will be to choose drugs that interact positively with a person's knowledge that he or she is a good person and that his own Altruistic Brain circuitry must now be allowed to operate. However, this is a hard problem. In prescribing with that principle in mind, doctors will encounter at least three difficulties: (1) drugs that had been thought to be specific to one neurochemical mechanism are not actually specific, (2) the therapist has no control over the time course of the drug's action, and (3) there will be huge individual differences (including sex differences) in responses to any given drug. Therefore, although some psychiatrists will recommend such pharmacotherapy, a great deal of data remains to be collected before we can ethically pursue this approach.

Popular sources in the media tend to discuss "talk therapy" as an alternative to drug therapy. Though there is an extensive literature on this question, it is clear that drug therapy alone is not sufficient. The combination of psychotherapy (a.k.a. talk therapy) with an optimized drug regimen is most likely to help a patient who already has committed serious antisocial acts. It is likely, therefore, that some combination of talk therapy and pharmacotherapy will best strengthen Altruistic Brain operations.

SOCIETY SHOULD REMOVE OBSTACLES TO LEADERSHIP BY WOMEN

Women's hormones, such as estrogen and oxytocin operating on circuits in the female brain, together with the neural systems they affect, foster prosocial attitudes and good behavior. Therefore, it is important to remove obstacles to women's participation in social leadership. Of course, there is no question that from an ethical perspective we cannot have a society in which one sex is subordinate to another; the point is that now, from a scientific perspective, it seems clear that we'd all be better off if women played a more and more prominent and vital role in civic life.

Indeed, a substantial body of opinion holds that if a greater proportion of leadership positions were occupied by women, the world would be more peaceful. According to these studies, carried out by psychologists in the United States and in Europe, there would be fewer wars, and less organized violence of any sort. Indeed, in women the Altruistic Brain's operations are exposed to less powerful hormonal opposition than they are in men. All of the biological forces for friendliness recounted in Chapter 5—oxytocin, estrogens, and other chemicals involved in mating and maternal behaviors—are in place in most women to help Altruistic Brain mechanisms work properly. Beyond simple maternal behavior, women have an interest in maintaining social stability, rather than up-ending it with war, as women are much more involved in raising children than are men. This is not a "cultural" observation, but a scientific fact. Reproductive biologists make clear that among primates, including *Homo sapiens*, women on average invest much more metabolic and physiological capital in the survival of their young than do men. Because primates' young are helpless for years, prolonged periods of social stability are valued by women acting as primary caregivers. Large-scale social turmoil, including war, is thus anathema to them, and they seek to avoid it.

Several books, articles, and websites have recently taken up this argument, contrasting men's and women's evolutionary biology, some of them offering detailed support for empowering women, as well as an array of practical, research-based approaches to avoiding violent conflict. They cite anthropological evidence for status-based factors that, on an enlarged scale, lead to war: "in male dominated societies, much of men's social lives revolve around rearranging the social order in their dominance hierarchies to achieve greater social status." Men want the comforts (what we might call "perks") that come with status, and are willing to fight to get it. The site notes that while the same impulse is found in women, it is "not as strongly expressed." In a similar vein, Joshua Goldstein argues in *War and Gender* that men may be more hierarchical—that is, oriented toward competition and status—whereas women are more empathetic, albeit with "a great deal of plasticity" in gender roles. Thus although there is some overlap between genders when it comes to aggressive tendencies, biologists and anthropologists concur that men display traits far more favorable to war.

Individual, somewhat surprising examples of how women cooperate are dramatic and easily illustrated. Consider pictures of Arab and Israeli women working together. In a symposium on preventing genocide, former Secretary of State Hillary Clinton suggested reaching out to women in potentially troubled areas; because women are averse to violence, they would be keenly sensitive to its impending outbreak and could provide an early warning to troubleshooters. At the elevated levels of world leadership in politics and finance, the ability of Christine Lagarde and Angela Merkel to move forward in a cooperative fashion is remarkable. Lagarde, the Managing Director of the International Monetary Fund, presses the larger and wealthier European countries to contribute to funds that will keep southern European countries from defaulting on their debts. In contrast, Merkel, Chancellor of Germany, tries to press southern European countries to reform their economic policies and pay their debts so that Germans do not end up supporting them. Despite their obviously different portfolios, however, these two women do not rip each other apart. They try to deal effectively with Europe's huge and continuing economic problems, and they are reported to remain friendly, sending each other texts and gifts. Of course, at this level of accomplishment there are not enough women to permit a scientific comparison with men. Nor would it be fair to assert that men cannot cooperate—they obviously can. But it does seem clear, indeed undeniable, that eliminating obstacles—ranging from duties in the home to educational inequalities to a lack of encouragement from family and friends—to women taking on more responsibility will serve the cause of non-confrontation and peace. Now we have seen the example of women senators, an astoundingly small minority, putting aside partisan differences to collectively promote a negotiated settlement to the 2013 government shutdown. As Senator Susan Collins observed, "I don't think it's a coincidence that women were so heavily involved in trying to end this stalemate. Although we span the ideological spectrum, we are used to working together in a collaborative way."

In parts of the world, we could not be further from the goal of empowering women. The continuing examples of degrading behaviors toward women tell us how far, as world citizens, we have to go to achieve the goal of empowering women worldwide. Tamara Kreinin, Executive Director for Women and Population at the United Nations Foundation has written about "violence against women, that has until recently, often remained hidden. It occurs primarily behind closed doors, in the presumed safe environment of the 'home' and in the hands of partners and other family members or acquaintances. Intimate partner violence and sexual violence against women, are the most common forms of violence that women experience." In some places, such violence is systematic, including genital mutilation and, more generally, violence that manifests itself as a historical problem born out of unequal power relations between men and women, and a lack of economic resources. The whole issue of violence against women in some countries can aptly be traced in the problems brought out by patriarchy as a cultural framework for gender relations. Women, whose neurochemistry more powerfully encourages altruistic behavior as detailed in Chapter 4, would, in this respect, provide better cultural leadership.

Thus in some of the world's 193 countries, the issue of empowering women addresses problems that are much worse than a typical middle-class situation in the United States. Education of women is of paramount importance, followed by providing enough economic support that they are not at the mercy of their countrymen.

Francis Fukuyama, professor of public policy at George Mason University, argues that "a world dominated completely by female leaders would be more peaceful than one where female leaders are in the minority." Of course, two objections immediately come to mind. First, it is easy to name belligerent female leaders such as Catherine the Great of Russia or England's Margaret Thatcher; it is even easier to name women who, like Golda Meir or Indira Gandhi, were willing to go to war. Second, if we reflect on Chapter 7, complex considerations of national policy by highly organized governments far exceed in their sophistication the knowledge that neuroscience can bring to bear regarding sex hormone effects on the brain. Thus we can cite any number of men—Dag Hammarskjold, Mahatma Ghandi, Martin Luther King, the Dalai Lama, Anwar Sadat, and an array of Sufi mystics—who fervently represent peace. Nevertheless, historically, men have indeed been more violent than women, and we do have testosterone's effects on the brain to contribute to that distinction.

While I want to avoid simple-minded extrapolations from sociobiology, to which Fukuyama seems susceptible, I do agree with him that "the basic social problem that any society faces is to control the aggressive tendencies of its young men." Put that problem together with Fukuyama's speculations and you reach the conclusion that, certainly, organizing societies so that women have an equal chance at attaining positions of power and influence has to be a good idea and that, on the average, women will be less willing to start wars or to pursue other violent policies. Of course, women have not held the reins of power nearly to the degree that men have. Only if women are enabled to assume positions of equal power will we know for sure how effective they are in keeping the peace. If "peace" is a strategic initiative—as to a degree it was for Egypt's Sadat and his Israeli counterpart, Itzhak Rabin—then women should be allowed to prove themselves in the strategic realm.

To empower women, the first step is education, along with helping young women to define career paths (e.g., as scientists or diplomats) that will allow Altruistic Brain operations their maximum social impact. In fact, neuroanatomical rationales that could support such policies—that is, that give weight to promoting women—are emerging from studies such as one performed by a group of Japanese scientists. They used magnetic resonance imaging to compare the brains of 66 young adult women with 89 men to test the "social brain hypothesis," which states that the expansion of the human (as opposed to nonhuman) brain was driven by the need for a tremendous amount of information processing to be used in social recognition and signaling. The scientists measured the volumes of the brain that contain nerve cell bodies, "gray matter," leaving out simple fiber tracts ("white matter") and dividing by body weight. Women had more gray matter, particularly in parts of the forebrain connected with social behavior. They inferred that women have more processing power in these "social brain" regions and correlated this with a greater capacity for altruistic, socially cooperative behaviors.

ROOM FOR HOPE

Given all the palliative measures at our disposal to address troubled individuals, as well as the potential for groups to pull more than their own weight, I cannot accept the view of those who foresee only decline for our country and indeed our species. Such ideas conjure up a sort of centrifugal momentum based on class warfare and the degradation of social norms, at odds with forces for cohesion and goodwill described in this book (and applied in this chapter in terms of an altruistic "multiplier" effect).

Consider, for example, Charles Murray's *Coming Apart*, which describes a fragmented American society in which distinct upper and lower classes can be identified on the basis of "core behaviors" and values, including attitudes toward family, vocation, community, and faith. But isn't this assessment just too neat? What about all of the cross-class phenomena—for example, suburban kids teaching in poor neighborhoods—that pull in the opposite direction? Moreover, even acknowledging this country's class distinctions, the prosocial behaviors made possible by Altruistic Brain mechanisms trump those distinctions. Think about the Robin Hood Foundation, or the Clinton and Gates Foundations—name-brand organizations that have their counterparts in literally hundreds more. No one *made* Bill Clinton or Bill Gates undertake initiatives that would reform schools and attack poverty. They just wanted to make a difference in terms of human welfare. Indeed, they were following the model of Andrew Carnegie, whose foundation still seeks to do "real and permanent good."

Nor is it just upper-class people who, through a sense of noblesse oblige, make efforts at bridging the wealth gap. Here is what American philanthropist Kim Hendler says about why she donates to the North Star Fund, a community foundation that supports grassroots groups leading the way toward "equality, economic justice, and peace":

My vision for the future: A New York City that's interconnected. I see people having more understanding and empathy for the challenges and assets that different groups of people bring to the table. I would like every New Yorker to have the opportunity to live in a safe place, to be able to access healthy food, to get a good education, and to have a voice in our political system.

For Ms. Hendler, it is not just the "City" that matters, but actual faces in the crowd. She tells the story of a child (also pictured) who must limp up three flights of stairs because war in his native country prevented his being vaccinated. Her anecdote brings to life the Altruistic Brain, the immediate empathy of one person for another that provokes that person to action. Hendler goes on to state that she believes that helping one another requires that we get out of our comfort zones, that we join forces with like-minded people to make a real difference: "Of course people need to be served a meal tonight because they're hungry. But it's also crucial to support work that's getting at the root cause of why so many people are hungry. It takes courage to take on a root cause because it requires us to evaluate the status quo and our roles—our comfort—in maintaining it." Hendler will "support work," that is, she will participate as part of a larger effort, so as to redress what she sees as class-based, degrading conditions. In wanting to root out these conditions by supporting the Fund, Hendler exemplifies the "multiplier" effect, invoking community as the sort of leveraging agent that Geoffery Canada envisions as well: "That's a set of values [tackling the root causes of poverty, shrugging off one's comfort] that I know I share with the rest of the North Star community, and why I am a part of it." I hope that the conservative American author Charles Murray, who wrote *The Bell Curve,* is listening. Ironically, while Charles Murray offers a generally pessimistic scenario, he sees as well the positive possibilities for social progress emanating from individuals' self-respect. This notion actually affirms the program put forward by James Gilligan, which has great potential for rectifying many of social ills that Murray himself predicts. We are led right back to the need for avoiding humiliation of the individual, especially early in life and most particularly with regard to young boys.

Any perception (real or conjectural) concerning American society's fragmentation must take neuroscience into account. If thinkers such as

Murray are going to worry about the shared "core" of our belief system, then how about the Golden Rule, which is built into the core of our neuroanatomy and knits us together through reciprocal morality. As illustrated in Chapter 1, stories of altruistic behavior crop up in the most unusual settings, even in those where anomie would seem to be a necessary condition of life. Think about US prisons, which in many cases are hugely overcrowded. Inmates with special needs may not be well served, even at the level acceptable for prisoners. Those with cognitive impairment pose special problems, and turn up more frequently than in the general population, perhaps because they have more risk factors, for example, head injuries. But here is the striking point: inmates, even killers, have been recruited successfully in a California prison to care for other inmates with Alzheimer's. They protect demented inmates from being robbed, escort them around the prison to keep them from getting lost, and help them to maintain personal hygiene. While the patients rarely say "thank you," these convicted killers still show compassion.

Laboratory experiments, often using "games," tell us that social cohesion and prosocial behavior are possible notwithstanding stressful conditions. Computer simulations demonstrate individuals' preference for *situational* cooperation even in populations whose constituents are so mobile that they fail to form strong, conventional social ties. In this regard, behavioral economists Carlos Roca and Dirk Helbing set up a simulation so that the moving "players" would refer only to their own experience and benefit when making decisions about social cooperation. On any given move, a player could cooperate (contribute) or not (defect). Given such choices, and the freedom to act according to their own advantage, players still chose cooperation—creating a type of social cohesion even under the stress of constant mobility.

Under many circumstances, good behavior spreads, such that "cascades" of cooperation are observable. A different set of social games set up under laboratory conditions by psychologists James

Fowler and Nicholas Christakis showed that the cooperative behaviors of people placed at the foci of social nets are influenced by what they observe from other game players; those observations influence such people as they behave toward still others who were not part of the initial interactions. Clearly, the feelings and welfare of one individual are of interest to others in the group, in the manner of a village. It does, indeed, "take a village." Over time, prosocial customs accumulate through instruction and imitation, such that the processes can be "ratcheted in complexity" in the words of Rachel Kendal.

Experiments with real human subjects reinforce and extend these conclusions. David Rand and his colleagues in the Program for Evolutionary Dynamics at Harvard recruited subjects to an incentivized economic game in which a player interacted with her neighbors, either cooperating (contributing) or defecting (not contributing). Crucially, before each decision in this game, each subject was reminded of all her neighbors' previous decisions. At the end of each turn each subject was informed about the decisions of her neighbors and her own payoff for that turn. Here was the bottom line: social networks were dynamic, and could even be "shuffled" by the experimenters such that neighborly relations did not remain constant. However, large-scale cooperation could be generated and maintained *if and only if* subjects could update their network connections frequently. When they did so, they formed links with cooperators and broke links with defectors. As a result of this dynamic, stable cooperation emerged.

Systematic scientific observations in many countries support an optimistic view regarding the possibility of cooperative behaviors even under difficult conditions. For example, in games conducted under an Agricultural Productivity Project for farmers in Uganda, individual and collective interests (e.g., regarding access to water and roads) were at odds. However, sociologists proved that a centralized, legitimate sanctioning power could still boost cooperative behavior. This game, as well as the others that I described, illustrates that prosocial behavior is achievable under adverse conditions—those that tend toward lack of cohesion—in much the same way that one would expect from societies that are highly integrated.

Other researchers reported an unusual experiment regarding the effects of ethno-religious diversity on human altruism. In Bosnia Herzegovina they studied the social behavior of Catholic Croats and Muslim Bosniaks in the same kind of public goods game mentioned above. In their game, all players decide simultaneously on what contributions they want to make to the common good, and after each round the sum is automatically increased by 20% and the public good equally divided among all players regardless of their contribution. When players came from segregated backgrounds, mixing them together reduced public good contributions and sanctions did not help. However, when players came from integrated backgrounds, mixing them together improved altruistic behavior, and adding a systematically devised, credible program of sanctions for selfish behavior increased public good contributions to their highest level. All of these different kinds of large group experiments show how, once an individual is convinced that he is both good and ethical, a variety of social tools and strategies can propel him into long-term, widespread cooperative relationships.

Several prominent primatologists have argued that our evolutionary history has yielded "man the warrior." But anthropologist Douglas Fry in his book *Beyond War* has reached the opposite conclusion, looking at the likely social behaviors of early humans by working with surviving tribes around the world. Based on ethnographic cases, he emphasizes "the human potential for peace." Also, consider the Waorani of Ecuador. Even though they are reputed to have "one of the most violent cultures on earth," years passed between raids and American anthropologists never actually saw a Waorani kill anyone. Likewise, the Mexican Zapotec tribe, in which there are indeed "periodic acts of physical aggression such as fist fights." However, most typical daily scenes are peaceful. For the Paliyan, a tribe in southern India, Fry notes that "hunting groups operate via discussion and consensus." They really do "live in accordance with a nonviolent ethos." He goes on to show the paucity of warfare among the aboriginal tribes in the Australian bush. In fact, "aboriginal Australians employed a rich set of social and legal mechanisms to resolve disputes within and among social groups." Fry's examples provide dramatic proof of humans' ability to live in peace, and "argue strongly against the belief that war is a natural attribute of humanity."

Anthropologist Raymond Kelly agrees with Fry's main point and adds characteristics of societies that get along without wars. These tend to be "unsegmented societies," "characterized by the minimal complement of social groups. They manifest only those social groups that are cultural universals, present in every society, and nothing more." I speculate that such societies permit individuals' Altruistic Brain mechanisms to operate unfettered.

Finally, Fry returns to the massively important, common sense argument exemplified in Chapter 1: "In actuality, the vast majority of the people on the planet awake on a typical morning and live through a violence-free day—and this experience generally continues day after day after day." This obvious fact reaffirms, from a different point of view, mechanisms for ABT described in Chapters 2 and 3 are actually working for the vast majority of the people, day after day.

I have been writing about neuronal circuits that dispose us all toward good behavior. Likewise, the social opportunities and challenges depicted here are likely true—at least to some degree—of every human society. We share the same Altruistic Brain mechanisms as well as many of the same social incentives to act morally. To encourage good behavior, therefore, societies should do what Harvard anthropology professor Ezra Vogel proposed would be necessary for the Chinese government to maintain credible authority: (1) provide universal social security and health care; (2) manage the boundaries of individual freedom to act, within the requirements for public order; (3) limit corruption; and (4) preserve the environment so that young people can imagine a safe future. Society must be safe and livable, with reliable and fair sanctions, so that people do not become disoriented or fall into such despair that they lose respect for themselves and trust in others. Both are necessary for optimal Altruistic Brain functioning, and for the "multiplier" effect that I have been describing to work.

PRACTICAL MEANS

So what are some of the practical means by which cooperative and even altruistic behaviors in society might be encouraged? In *SuperCooperators*, Nowak spells out his ideas about "mechanics of cooperation:"

- Repetition and foreknowledge that repeated interactions can be expected. During the Prisoner's Dilemma computer game (see Chapter 3), the success of simple programs that proved to be "evolutionary stable strategies" depended on repetition.
- One's ethical behavior toward another will be encouraged by one's impression that this other will behave kindly toward one in return.
- Network formation. It will always be true that some individuals will interact socially more than others. Key to this will be the formation of social clusters that help each other, with the limiting condition that the benefit-to-cost ratio of joining the cluster must be seen by the new "joiner" as adequate.
- More than one level of social interaction determines cooperation. Nowak means that computer-program cooperation

evolved best if substantial numbers of groups and levels of groups are involved in the process of developing cooperative behaviors, not just individuals.

We can practice these principles, supported by knowledge that our brains are designed to make them work and to make them eminently practicable on a day-to-day basis.

In fact, the transition from ideal to practicable has already begun, as the practical applicability of ABT is now recognized in the literature. In "Reciprocity and Neuroscience in Public Health Law" (2011), an article written after he heard me lecture, the bioethicist A. M. Viens examines how the theory could assist public health officials in managing an emergency. I quote an extended passage, as it conveys just how practical the theory's possibilities are:

Extending this [theory] to the context of public health and the case of quarantine, one possibility is that individuals may have a tendency to avoid performing harmful acts—the consequences of which they themselves would fear. For non-infected individuals, this may mean motivation to undertake testing and adequate precautions, reporting exposed individuals breaking quarantine, among other considerations. For healthcare professionals, this may mean motivation to fulfill their duty to care in the face of increased risk and conflicting personal obligations to family. Even for infected individuals, who may have fallen victim to the consequences they feared, this still may mean motivation to cooperate with isolation measures, being compliant with treatment, taking active steps not to expose or infect others. For government and public health officials, this may mean provision of the necessities of life....

Notice how often this analysis uses the term "motivation." From Viens' perspective, ABT provides public officials with a rationale for *encouraging* actors in a crisis to act responsibly, based on such officials' *knowledge* that they will likely do so. Rather than forcing people to act according to publically desirable norms, the measures outlined by Viens gain force from people's own desire to prevent consequences that they would not wish to suffer themselves. The effect is to enlist people in a public effort by relying on their own good will. Writ large, Viens provides a template for all sorts of emergencies—not just public health—and indeed for all sorts of undertakings requiring a unified, multipronged response where those who are and are not damaged must each play a part. This is why his approach is exciting.

Viens goes on to observe that the success of any such "motivational" measures depends on explaining them, on getting word out to affected constituencies that the generous response is actually beneficial: "[P]ublic health laws involving restrictive measures (author's note, like not smoking in restaurants and not consuming diabetes-inducing sugary drinks in large amounts) could make use of this neurobiological predisposition to reciprocate by ensuring that individuals doing their part are adequately supported and assisted in fulfilling their obligations, and [that] concrete estimations of the benefits and burdens are accurately communicated to assure everyone that the balance of benefit over harm is highly favorable." If people *know* that reciprocal morality benefits the entire community, they will most likely act morally. *The Altruistic Brain* is intended to help make such knowledge available and comprehensible.

Indeed, it attempts to provide a new, more circuit-specific framework for emerging interest in the brain's altruistic inclinations. In an analysis of recent work on the effect of neuroscience on law, Edwin Scott Fruehwald observed that such work describes a "theory of biology," in which "reciprocal altruism antedates formal institutions, and . . . appears to be hard-wired into human brains. In other words, there is a universal grammar of reciprocity just like there is a universal grammar of language." Scientists are beginning to sense that humans possess mechanisms that propel them towards altruism, and are using the language of computers and linguistics to convey this understanding. Now they can use the language of the brain itself. We can now show how the brain *actually* operates to produce good behavior.

OUTLOOK

Starting from the assumption that we no longer need to speak in terms of analogy and metaphor when describing the brain's altruistic mechanisms, this book seeks to launch an inquiry into altruism from an understanding of *exactly* how we act well toward each other. Many influential thinkers see big trouble ahead for modern human society: overpopulation, water shortages, terrorism, nuclear proliferation, energy shortages, underemployment, and the like. Consider our capacity for survival. In 1962, during Premier Nikita Khruschev's reign in Moscow and John F. Kennedy's presidency, with Russian ships steaming toward an American blockade of Cuba's nuclear missile–bearing island, these two men headed off a nuclear confrontation. Our need to survive prevailed, and these leaders figured out how. Neither man wanted to hurt his country, or others. No doubt the same has been true during less publicized episodes. I hope that we can begin to forge a new understanding of our species as we seek to continue to survive. I do not concur in Sylvia Nasar's wish that our species' Latin designation change from *Homo sapiens* to *Homo ethicus*, but I do think that the vitality of our brain's moral circuitry should be acknowledged to be better than in some quarters is casually assumed.

It is important that we recognize the brain's moral proclivities, because doing so actually strengthens those proclivities. As I have argued, good character is in part the product of a powerful feedback loop: when we think better of ourselves, we try to live up to that self-estimation. In effect, if we think that we can be good members of society, we do not want to disappoint ourselves, potentially falling back into despair. Thus in this book I have tried to demonstrate just how plausible our own built-in kindness actually is, how scientifically reasonable it can be to *rely* on the idea that we are wired from infancy to "do the right thing." If the altruism built into the human brain becomes more plausible on account of our scientific understanding, then there is genuine cause for optimism notwithstanding all of our continuing challenges.

FURTHER READING

M. Bazerman and A. Tenbrunsel. 2012. *Blind Spots*. Princeton, NJ: Princeton University Press.

W. T. Boyce. 2004. "Social Stratification, Health and Violence in the Very Young." *Annals of the New York Academy of Sciences* 1036, 47–68.

J. Devine, ed. 2004. "Youth Violence: Scientific Approaches to Prevention." *Annals of the New York Academy of Sciences* 1036, 13–46.

Douglas Fry. 2007. *Beyond War*. Oxford: Oxford University Press.

Francis Fukuyama. 1998. "Women and the Evolution of World Politics." *Foreign Affairs* 77, 24–40.

James Gilligan. 2001. *Preventing Violence*. London: Thames and Hudson.

Mark Greenberg. 2010. "School-based Prevention: Current Status and Future Challenges." *Effective Education* 2, 27–52.

Daniel Kahneman. 2011. *Thinking Fast and Slow*. New York: Macmillan.

Daniel Kahneman and Amos Tversky. 2000. *Choices, Values and Frames*. Cambridge: Cambridge University Press.

Raymond Kelly. *Warless Societies and the Origin of War*. Ann Arbor: University of Michigan Press.

D. Kennedy. 2012. *Don't Shoot: One Man, a Street Fellowship, and the End of Violence in Inner-city America*. London: Bloomsbury.

Sylvia Nasar. 2011. *Grand Pursuit: The Story of Economic Genius*. New York: Simon & Schuster.

Martin Nowak. 2012. *SuperCooperators*. New York: Simon & Schuster.

Doanld Pfaff. 2011. *Man and Woman: An Inside Story*. New York: Oxford University Press.

Stephen Post. 2007. *Why Good Things Happen to Good People*. New York: Alfred A. Knopf.

K. Schenck-Gustafsson. 2012. *Gender Medicine*. Zurich: Karger.

H. Yamasue, O. Abe, M. Suga, H. Yamada, M. A. Rogers, S. Aoki, N. Kato, and K. Kasai. 2008. "Sex-linked Neuroanatomical Basis of Human Altruistic Cooperativeness." *Cerebral Cortex* 18, 2331–2340.

INDEX

Page numbers followed by the italicized letter *f* indicate material found in figures.